#ChickenSoup
Old Remedy, New Again

Written by Sheldon Yakiwchuk
Cover by Gary Sweitzer

All rights reserved.

ISBN: 978-1-7381434-0-5

All rights reserved, including the right to reproduce this book, or portions thereof, in any form. No part of this book may be reproduced, scanned, or distributed in any printed or electronic form without permission. For permission requests, write to the publisher.

Sheldon Yakiwchuk

Old Remedy, New Again.

Disclaimer:

This book, #ChickenSoup is authored by Sheldon Yakiwchuk, who is not a medical doctor or licensed healthcare professional. The information provided in this book is intended for general educational and informational purposes only. It is not intended as a substitute for professional medical advice, diagnosis, or treatment.

The content within this book is based on the author's personal research, experiences, and opinions, as well as information available up to the date of publication. Nutritional science and health guidelines may evolve, and it is essential to consult with a qualified healthcare provider or registered dietitian before making significant dietary or lifestyle changes, starting a new nutritional plan, or addressing specific health concerns.

Readers are encouraged to seek the guidance of a licensed healthcare professional for personalized recommendations tailored to their individual health status, medical history, and specific dietary needs. Any reliance on the information presented in this book is at the reader's discretion and risk.

The author and publisher of Sheldon Yakiwchuk do not assume responsibility for any errors, inaccuracies, or omissions in the content, or for any adverse effects, consequences, or outcomes resulting from the use or application of the information provided herein. Individual results may vary, and no specific outcomes are guaranteed.

Readers are advised to use their judgment and discretion when applying any nutritional or dietary information from this book. It is recommended to consult with a healthcare professional for any medical concerns or questions related to nutritional choices and their impact on health.

By reading this book, you acknowledge and agree to the terms of this disclaimer and understand that the author and publisher are not liable for any actions or decisions made based on the content of this publication.

Contents

Acknowledgements
Introduction
Preface
Hippocratic Oath
Preamble and Ingredients
Vitamins, Minerals and Nutrients
Preamble Amino Acids
Vitamin, Minerals and Nutrient Benefits
Amino Acid Benefits
Summary of Benefits
Preamble on Fillers
COVID
Immune Triggers and Immune Energy
Sarcopenia
Cachexia
Summary and recap on Immune Triggers and Immune Energy
Thermogenesis
Thermogenesis Summary
Soup or Broth?
Less is More
Correlative Analysis
Back to when Less is More
Fasting
Keto Flu
Conclusion

Old Remedy, New Again.

Acknowledgements

To say that the depths of information presented were any of my own work would simply be disingenuous. In truth, while I've spent countless hours researching information brought out by some of the nutritional giants and low-carb advocates, pouring over medical studies and journals, learning about the functions of nutrition, benefits to the body and metabolism, the information here is merely assembled off the dedication and efforts of others.

This book's creation was a team effort that benefited from the assistance, direction, and inspiration of numerous sources.

I also want to express my gratitude to the academics, teachers, and other professionals whose knowledge and viewpoints served as the basis for this book's content. Your contributions to a variety of academic subjects have improved the knowledge on these pages.

To the YakkStack Community who has continued to provide unwavering support, encouragement, patience and acceptance of my continuous grammatical and punctuation errors, your replies and comments have meant everything to me and have encouraged me to finally take my first steps in the world of book writing.

Old Remedy, New Again.

Introduction

Few recipes are as beloved and revered as chicken soup in the world of comfort food. Touted as a cure-all for both physical and mental ills, it is a culinary tradition that has been passed down through the years, whispered from grandmothers to grandchildren. Whether relished as a comforting dinner on a frigid winter evening or as a hearty treatment for the common cold, chicken soup has gone beyond simple feeding to become a symbol of warmth, healing, and nourishment.

But chicken soup is more than just a warm bowl of broth with some vegetables and chicken in it. A nutritional powerhouse with a symphony of vitamins, minerals, and other bioactive components hides beneath the seemingly straightforward exterior. These substances not only satisfy the palate but also have a number of positive health effects.

We will learn the truths behind this liquid gold's lore as a healing potion as we delve into its depths. We'll examine the vitamins and minerals that make it a nutrient-rich treasure trove, analyze how its components affect our immune system, and find out how it may calm our souls just as well as our sore throats. What you want altered should go here. After that, click the button below. It's that simple!

Join me on this medical journey, where we'll discuss the traditional knowledge that has been passed down through the ages as well as the cutting-edge research that supports the notion that chicken soup has healing properties. The nutritional miracles contained in a boiling pot of chicken and broth—a culinary joy that transcends time, borders, and, most importantly, the boundaries of good health—will enlighten, inspire, and, of course, tempt you.

Welcome to the nutritional world of chicken soup!

Old Remedy, New Again.

Preface

Do you remember when we used to treat sniffles with Chicken Soup and not pure fascism?

This is a question that I've both come across and asked myself quite often in respect to COVID, with the Vaccinations, Mandates, other Non-Pharmaceutical Interventions (NPIs) and all of the dubious health advice that we've all been witness to over the last 4 years. Coming into another Respiratory Virus Season of what will most likely be pure panic, additional vaccinations (Influenza and COVID), mask wearing…I figured I'd take some time to dive into the Chicken Soup side of things, to perhaps offer an alternate and yet age-old perspective.

To give an idea of how far this goes back, Hippocrates, Father of Western Medicine (Hippocratic Oath), who coined the phrase, "Let food be thy medicine", prescribed a version of Chicken Soup to his patients as a treatment for respiratory illnesses in the 5th century BCE.

Hippocratic Oath:

I swear by Apollo the physician, and Asclepius, and Hygieia and Panacea and all the gods and goddesses as my witnesses, that, according to my ability and judgment, I will keep this Oath and this contract:

To hold him who taught me this art equally dear to me as my parents, to be a partner in life with him, and to fulfill his needs when required; to look upon his offspring as equals to my own siblings, and to teach them this art, if they shall wish to learn it, without fee or contract; and that by the set rules, lectures, and every other mode of instruction, I will impart a knowledge of the art to my own sons, and those of my teachers, and to students bound by this contract and having sworn this Oath to the law of medicine, but to no others.

I will use those dietary regimens which will benefit my patients according to my greatest ability and judgment, and I will do no harm or injustice to them.

I will not give a lethal drug to anyone if I am asked, nor will I advise such a plan; and similarly, I will not give a woman a pessary to cause an abortion.

In purity and according to divine law will I carry out my life and my art.

I will not use the knife, even upon those suffering from stones, but I will leave this to those who are trained in this craft.

Into whatever homes I go, I will enter them for the benefit of the sick, avoiding any voluntary act of impropriety or corruption, including the seduction of women or men, whether they are free men or slaves.

Whatever I see or hear in the lives of my patients, whether in connection with my professional practice or not, which ought not to be spoken of outside, I will keep secret, as considering all such things to be private.

So long as I maintain this Oath faithfully and without corruption, may it be granted to me to partake of life fully and the practice of my art, gaining the respect of all men for all time. However, should I transgress this Oath and violate it, may the opposite be my fate.

If only this oath was still treated according to the spirit it was written.

It's special thanks to the Internet that we are now in the true age of information but the problems with this being, our time is limited, and the information is exhaustingly overabundant, unclear, and often conflicting. Almost every week you will find an article online, in a magazine or newspaper about how eggs are good for you, preceded by the following week, the same sources reporting on how bad they are. Coffee? Same, and there really is no shortage of examples.

It's not so different from demonizing processed meats due to them using nitrates in curing or processing. "Don't eat cold cuts, bacon or hotdogs, because they contain nitrates", they all screech. But what about the nitrates in unprocessed natural foods like celery, raw spinach or beets?

Are the nitrates in spinach as bad as the nitrates in a hotdog?

[Blank stare…eyes blinking unknowingly], is what you can as a reply, if you were to ask this question.

No wonder that people have seemingly tapped out on reading up on diets and nutrition and why obesity is rampant in the westernized world. It's just too damned confusing!

Add to this, healthy foods have become increasingly more expensive, fast foods have been cost effective, a lot found on dollar menus in your favorite fast-food chain. No prep required. No dishes to be done. A few bucks in and shazam, you're fed.

Packaged food items are no better and it's not like the manufacturers/providers of these foods are doing their best to keep people informed. They use small portions of their products as if this somehow proves benefits and to help keep the eyeline away from the actual ingredients. As an example, potato chips give a rating per 20 chips to say, "See, these aren't so bad", full well knowing that nobody is out there calculating their way through a full bag, counting how many chips they've eaten, nor trying to figure out how many calories are in the crumbs at the bottom of the bag. Items like chips, cookies, sugar coated breakfast cereals even having a section of the packaging that states, 'Nutritional Facts' on them is purely offensive.

Even prior to 2020, you'd most likely already heard that having chicken soup was good for a cold, or even if you are just cold, and without even realizing how far back this dates. You might even have your own specific recipes or books of recipes on it. Like everything else on the internet, there is no shortage of information.

If you googled "chicken soup", you'll find 800+ Million results.

If you googled "chicken soup recipes", almost a Billion results…which seems a little crazy, since all you're doing is adding the word "recipes", and you get an additional 200 million results.

And, if you want to see if Chicken Soup has ever been scientifically studied for benefits, PubMed has 215 of its own results. Truth be known, while I've only read a few of these studies, they talk about the effects of Chicken Soup, they don't really answer the questions as to How or Why it may produce benefits.

This is where and how confusion can come into play. Clicking your way through trying to figure this out, you're more likely to end up seeing websites on cat pictures or polar bears, forgetting what you were even looking for when you first started looking and then just ordering some Skip, because you don't even feel like making soup anymore.

It's like the intentional dumbing down of society so that you will just follow instructions and never really understand anything.

The proverbial, "take 2 of these and call me in the morning", ad nauseam, perpetually and indefinitely until mortality.

There's really not much point in analyzing why this is happening or getting into the conspiracy theories, when I'd just set out to provide you with some information on soup.

Anyways, let's get on with the soup!

Starting with the Ingredients.

The first thing I will say about the ingredients is that I am not going to provide a recipe and I am not going to argue about whose grandma/oma/baba makes a better soup. What I am going to do is go through the list of common ingredients, as we would have seen in traditional, Centuries-Old versions and break these down to their healing properties.

The basis for a good soup is the broth, where if you have a terrible broth, you're going to have a terrible soup. With this being said, when you have a cold, flu or even COVID, two of the identifiers of these respiratory illnesses can be anosmia (loss of smell) and ageusia (loss of taste) and may lead you to believing that this becomes less important. This is not the case at all because even if you do suffer from these conditions and your taster isn't quite up to snuff, you're still going to want to focus on what goes inside of your broth and the benefits they can provide.

Ingredients:

Main:
Chicken - Whole
Water
Vegetables:
Carrots
Celery
Onions
Garlic
Herbs and Spices:

Parsley
Thyme
Oregano
Basil
Bay leaves
Turmeric
Salt
Black Pepper

All of these?

Well, maybe…maybe not, you decide what you add to your version, I'm just going to break them down for you to let you know that none of these are accidental ingredients nor do they only serve a single purpose.

I'm not going to spend a lot of time on why you need to add water to your soup, with the exception of saying that if you didn't, you wouldn't have soup. One of the main benefits of having soup is the hydrating nature of soup and this in itself is important enough.

Vitamins, Minerals and Nutrients

Chicken: Vitamins A, B3, B6, B9, B12, D, Amino Acids, Choline, Creatine, Copper, Iron, Magnesium, Phosphorus, Potassium, Selenium, Zinc.

Chicken Bones: Collagen, Gelatin, Calcium, Magnesium, Phosphorus, Potassium, Glycosaminoglycans, Glucosamine, Glycine, Proline.

Chicken Skin: Vitamin E, Phosphorus, Potassium, Collagen.

Carrots: Vitamins A, B6, C, E, K1, Iron, Magnesium, Potassium, Calcium, Sodium.

Celery: Vitamins A, B6, B9, C, Calcium, Copper, Iron, K, Magnesium, Molybdenum, Phosphorus, Sodium.

Onions: Vitamins A, B6, B9, C, Allicin, Copper, Folate, Iron, Manganese, Potassium, Quercetin.

Parsley: Vitamins A, B6, B9, C, K, Calcium, Copper, Iron, Manganese, Potassium.

Garlic: Vitamins B6, C, Allicin, Calcium, Choline, Copper, Folate, Iron, Manganese, Phosphorus, Potassium, Selenium.

.

Thyme: Vitamins A, B6, B9, C, K, Calcium, Copper, Iron, Potassium, Sodium.

Oregano: Vitamins A, B6, C, K, Calcium, Copper, Iron, Manganese, Potassium.

Basil: Vitamins A, B6, C, E, K, Calcium, Copper, Iron, Magnesium, Manganese, Potassium, Sodium.

Bay leaves: Vitamins A, C, B6, B9, Calcium, Potassium, Iron, Magnesium, Manganese, Zinc

Turmeric: Vitamins B6, C, E, Calcium, Copper, Curcumin, Iron, Manganese, Phosphorous, Potassium, Selenium, Zinc.

Black Pepper: Vitamins, B6, C, K, Calcium, Copper, Iron, Manganese, Potassium, Magnesium, Sodium, Piperine, Protein.

The total vitamin and nutrient profile of these ingredients is: Vitamins A, B3, B6, B9, B12, C, E, K, K1, Allicin, Calcium, Choline, Copper, Curcumin, Iron, Magnesium, Manganese, Molybdenum, Phosphorous, Piperine, Potassium, Quercetin, Selenium, Zinc.

From the previous lists of vitamins, minerals, and nutrients there are a lot of crossovers, much the reason that I said that you can decide which of the ingredients from the list that you'd prefer and which you can leave out.

Now, if you compared the profile of Vitamins on this list, you'd see that you essentially have the equivalent of a multivitamin, in a delicious fluid form. This is important because have you ever accidentally bit into a multivitamin or had one caught in your throat?

It's disgusting. It tastes like you threw up, inside of your mouth.

And then, If you compared the profile of a broth just made with the previously listed ingredients, to electrolytic sports beverages, what you'd notice is that you have a more complete electrolyte profile, a lot more essential vitamins, no added sugars, artificial flavors and coloring agents whose only profile is for coloring. In the Classic Versions of Chicken soup - predominantly yellow broth, gets this natural coloring from the turmeric.

I'm not saying whip up a batch of soup and pour it into your water bottle to take with you to the tennis court, soccer field or out on a bike ride. Cold Soup is gross, and the vegetables are bound to clog up your drinking spout. The importance of mentioning this is to say that keeping properly hydrated throughout a bout of illness is a great advantage in not adding the symptoms of dehydration.

In addition to just the vitamins, nutrients and minerals, Chicken is loaded with amino acids and their specific importance cannot be overstated, when it comes to the possible healing benefits of a bowl of Chicken Soup.

Chicken - Amino Acid Profile: Arginine, Cysteine, Glycine, Histidine, Isoleucine, Leucine, Lysine, Methionine, Phenylalanine, Proline, Serine, Threonine, Tryptophan, Valine.

And in this Amino Acid Profile, all 9 of the Essential Amino Acids are present - Histidine, Isoleucine, Leucine, Methionine, Phenylalanine, Threonine, Tryptophan, Valine. Essential Amino Acids being organic compounds that our body requires to function. These listed are deemed Essential because they are not amino acids that our bodies can produce and must come from consumption.

Addition to this, all 3 of the Branched-Chain Amino Acids (BCAAs) are represented - Leucine, Isoleucine, and Valine. BCAAs stimulate the building of proteins in muscle and have the ability to reduce muscle breakdown - I'll be going over why this is of particular importance later on.

Addition to Essentials, and BCAAs, Chicken not only contains Creatine, but also contains the 3 Amino Acids that are the building blocks of Creatine - Arginine, Glycine and Methionine - I'll also be going over why this is of particular importance later on.

And while I could assemble information on the benefits of each of the Amino Acids into a complete book of its own, I'm going to rein it in, keep to high points and just mention one more significant thing about the one of the Amino Acids - Leucine. When Leucine breaks down, it gets broken down into HydroxyMethylButyrate - HMB.

On purpose, I've waited until now to list all of the benefits of the previously listed Vitamins and nutrients. There is a lot to it and you may already know what they do and you can skim or skip the next several pages of me listing their individual benefits or just look up the ones you don't know.

Addition to this, if you don't fully understand everything that is listed by way of these benefits, don't worry. After having studied this for several years, a lot of the sciency type words and processes, I am not entirely sure of what it all means – excepting of the fact that I can appreciate these as benefits.

Do what I do.

Skim through, absorb what you can, nod your head knowingly and move on.

There are a lot of benefits listed that I don't fully cover because they aren't necessarily specific to the idea behind immune support by way of their function. While all of these processes do support immunity in some way, if I included them all, this book would be 7000 pages, nobody would read it and it'd be worthless.

Vitamin, Mineral and Nutrient Benefits

Vitamin A:

Vision: Vitamin A is crucial for good vision, especially when it comes to low light situations. It is a part of the retinal protein rhodopsin, which aids in night vision. Night blindness and, in severe situations, total blindness can result from a vitamin A deficiency.

Immune System Support: Vitamin A helps to keep the immune system in good shape. White blood cells, which are crucial for battling infections, are produced by the body with its assistance. A robust immune response depends on adequate vitamin A levels.

Skin Health: Vitamin A plays a crucial role in preserving healthy skin. It promotes skin cell growth and regeneration, reduces dryness and flakiness, and promotes a young appearance. Vitamin A derivatives can be found in some topical lotions and treatments for skin disorders.

Cell Growth and Differentiation: Vitamin A plays a role in controlling cell division and growth. It aids in ensuring normal cell growth and operation. This is crucial in tissues like the skin and mucous membranes that have a quick cell turnover.

Reproductive Health: Both males and females need vitamin A for healthy reproduction. It contributes to sperm production and supports the healthy growth of the placenta in females during pregnancy.

Antioxidant Activity: Beta-carotene, which is a precursor of vitamin A, has antioxidant properties. It aids in defending cells against injury from dangerous chemicals known as free radicals, which are connected to several chronic diseases and aging.

Bone Health: By promoting the growth and maintenance of bone cells, vitamin A contributes to sustaining bone health.

Cellular Communication: Vitamin A participates in the signaling and communication processes within cells. It aids in the normal functioning of cells and their response to outside signals.

Maintenance of Mucous Membranes: The mucous membranes that line the ocular, respiratory, gastrointestinal, and urinary systems benefit from vitamin A's ability to support their health. This maintains healthy function and works to prevent infections.

B3:

Energy Metabolism: The metabolism of carbohydrates, lipids, and proteins requires the coenzyme vitamin B3. It aids the body's transformation of these macronutrients into utilizable energy.

DNA Repair and Synthesis: Vitamin B3 is essential for DNA synthesis and repair. It contributes to the preservation of the genomic integrity of cells.

Cell Signaling: Niacin has a role in several cellular signaling events in its coenzyme form. It contributes to the normal operation of the nervous system and other physiological functions by assisting in the transmission of messages within and between cells.

Skin Health: Niacin may benefit the condition of your skin. It is incorporated into skincare products to help with skin appearance, inflammation reduction, and disorders like acne.

Cholesterol Regulation: Niacin has been demonstrated to have a positive impact on blood lipid levels in terms of regulating cholesterol. Low-density lipoprotein (LDL, or "bad" cholesterol), triglycerides, and high-density lipoprotein (HDL, or "good" cholesterol) can all be decreased by it. As a result, niacin is a component of various drugs that decrease cholesterol.

Cardiovascular Health: Niacin may help lower the risk of cardiovascular disorders, such as heart disease and atherosclerosis (hardening of the arteries), because of its capacity to enhance lipid profiles.

Anti-Inflammatory Effects: Niacin contains anti-inflammatory qualities and could aid in reducing inflammation in the body. Heart disease and several autoimmune disorders are two ailments that are linked to chronic inflammation.

Mental Health: Niacin intake should be adequate for maintaining mental health. Pellagra symptoms, which include dermatitis, diarrhea, dementia, and other neuropsychiatric signs and symptoms, can be brought on by a niacin shortage.

Digestive Health: Niacin promotes digestive health by assisting with food metabolism and nutrient absorption in the gastrointestinal tract.

Neurotransmitter Production: Niacin is involved in the manufacture of neurotransmitters, such as serotonin, which is important for mood regulation and emotional stability.

DNA Methylation: Niacin participates in DNA methylation, which controls gene expression and has an impact on a variety of biological processes.

Vitamin B6:

Metabolism: The metabolism of carbohydrates, proteins, and lipids depends on vitamin B6. It aids in transforming these macronutrients into energy the body may use for a variety of processes.

Brain Development and Function: Vitamin B6 is essential for appropriate brain function throughout life and for the formation of the developing brain in babies. It contributes to the synthesis of neurotransmitters, which are chemical messengers that carry signals throughout the brain.

Red Blood Cell Formation: Hemoglobin, a protein found in red blood cells that transports oxygen to bodily tissues, needs vitamin B6 to be made. Anemia can result from a vitamin B6 deficiency.

Immune System Support: Support for the Immune System: Vitamin B6 aids in the body's production of antibodies, which are proteins that assist the body fight off diseases and infections.

Nervous System Health: Health of the Nervous System: Vitamin B6 aids in the maintenance of the nervous system's health in addition to its function in the synthesis of neurotransmitters. It aids in the transfer of nerve signals and can lessen the symptoms of ailments like carpal tunnel syndrome.

Hormone Regulation: Vitamin B6 plays a role in the control of hormones, particularly those that affect mood and sleep. Premenstrual syndrome (PMS) symptoms may be lessened, and it may also promote emotional well-being.

Amino Acid Metabolism: The breakdown and usage of amino acids, which are the building blocks of proteins, depends on vitamin B6. As the body requires, it aids in the conversion of one amino acid into another.

Glycogen Breakdown: Vitamin B6 has a role in the breakdown of glycogen, which is used to store glucose in the muscles and liver. When needed, this procedure offers a rapid source of energy.

Skin Health: Vitamin B6 helps to maintain healthy skin by helping to make collagen, a protein that promotes the structure and elasticity of the skin.

Homocysteine Regulation: Vitamin B6, in addition to other B vitamins like folate and B12, aids in the control of blood homocysteine levels. The risk of cardiovascular disease is raised by elevated homocysteine levels.

Vitamin B9:

DNA Synthesis and Repair: One of vitamin B9's main activities is its role in the creation and repair of DNA, the genetic material found in cells. This is crucial for healthy cell division and development, making it crucial during times of fast growth like pregnancy and infancy.

Cell Division and Tissue Growth: Vitamin B9 is crucial for cell division and the growth and development of tissues, including those of the developing fetus during pregnancy. Adequate folate intake is critical for preventing neural tube defects in infants.

Red Blood Cell Formation: Folate is required for the formation of red blood cells, which transport oxygen throughout the body. Anemia, which is characterized by weakness, exhaustion, and pale complexion, can result from a folate shortage.

Homocysteine Regulation: Vitamin B9, along with other B vitamins like B6 and B12, aids in controlling blood levels of homocysteine. The risk of cardiovascular disease is raised by elevated homocysteine levels.

Brain and Nervous System Function: Folate contributes to the synthesis of neurotransmitters and supports healthy brain and nervous system function. For proper mood control and cognitive function, a person needs to consume enough folate.

Prevention of Birth Defects: Enough folate should be consumed, especially in the first trimester of pregnancy, to protect growing babies from neural tube defects like spina bifida.

Treatment of Certain Anemias: Folate is used to treat certain anemias, including megaloblastic anemia, which is characterized by unusually large and undeveloped red blood cells.

Support for Skin and Hair Health: Vitamin B9 helps with cell growth and repair, which results in healthy skin and hair.

Immune System Function: Folate is involved in immune system function and can support the body's ability to fend off diseases and infections.

Digestive Health: Vitamin B9 promotes a healthy digestive system and supports healthy digestion.

Vitamin B12:

Red Blood Cell Formation: The generation of red blood cells in the bone marrow depends on vitamin B12. Hemoglobin, the protein that delivers oxygen in red blood cells, is created with its help. Megaloblastic anemia, which results in bigger and fewer red blood cells that can't function properly, causes exhaustion and weakness, can be brought on by a vitamin B12 shortage.

Nervous System Function: Vitamin B12 is necessary for the healthy operation of the neurological system. It contributes to the preservation of the myelin sheath, which surrounds nerve cells as a protective layer. Neurological symptoms such as tingling, numbness, and poor coordination can result from a vitamin B12 shortage.

DNA Synthesis: Vitamin B12 is necessary for cell division and DNA synthesis. It is crucial for cells that divide quickly, like those in the gastrointestinal system and bone marrow.

Energy Metabolism: The metabolism of proteins, lipids, and carbohydrates is regulated by vitamin B12.

It aids in the body's ability to transform these macronutrients into usable energy.

Homocysteine Regulation: Folate and vitamin B12 work together to convert the amino acid homocysteine into the amino acid methionine. The risk of developing cardiovascular disease is raised by high blood homocysteine levels. Consuming enough vitamin B12 can help control homocysteine levels.

Cell Growth and Division: Vitamin B12 is necessary for all bodily cell growth and division, including the growth of skin, hair, and nail cells.

Supports Cognitive Function: Maintaining adequate levels of vitamin B12 may assist promote cognitive function and lower the risk of cognitive decline, including dementia, in older persons, according to some research.

Vitamin C:

Antioxidant Activity: Vitamin C has strong antioxidant properties that help shield cells from damage brought on by free radicals. Oxidative stress, which is associated to a number of chronic diseases and the aging process, can be brought on by free radicals, which are unstable molecules.

Immune System Support: Vitamin C is necessary for a healthy immune system. White blood cell formation and function, which are essential for battling infections, are stimulated. The severity and length of colds and other illnesses can be decreased by consuming enough vitamin C.

Collagen Production: Collagen is a structural protein that is crucial for the health of the skin, blood vessels, tendons, ligaments, and bones. Vitamin C is required for the synthesis of collagen. Collagen aids in wound healing and gives tissues strength and flexibility.

Skin Health: Vitamin C is crucial for keeping healthy skin because it aids in the formation of collagen and has antioxidant qualities. It can help lessen the appearance of wrinkles and fine lines as well as shield the skin from UV radiation damage.

Wound Healing: Vitamin C is essential for both tissue repair and wound healing. As part of the healing process, it aids the body in producing fresh skin, connective tissue, and blood vessels.

Iron Absorption: Vitamin C improves the digestive system's ability to absorb nonheme iron, which is the form of iron included in plant-based diets. Iron deficiency anemia can be avoided in this way, especially in people who eat vegetarian or vegan diets.

Eye Health: Vitamin C may help lower the risk of age-related macular degeneration and cataracts, two disorders of the eyes that are frequently associated with vision loss.

Stress reduction: According to some research, vitamin C may help lessen the negative psychological and physical impacts of stress.

Heart Health: A sufficient consumption of vitamin C is linked to a lower risk of heart disease. It could enhance blood vessel health, lower inflammation, and lower blood pressure.

Antiviral and Antimicrobial Effects: Vitamin C has demonstrated some antiviral and antibacterial characteristics that may aid the body in battling illnesses.

Cancer Prevention: While more research is required, several studies indicate that vitamin C may help lower the chance of developing some cancers. This may be because vitamin C has antioxidant characteristics and helps repair DNA.

Brain Health: Neurotransmitters like serotonin and norepinephrine, which can alter mood and cognitive function, are produced because of vitamin C.

Vitamin E:

Antioxidant Activity: Vitamin E has powerful antioxidant properties that help shield cells from damage brought on by free radicals. Free radicals are inherently unstable substances that can cause oxidative stress and harm to DNA, proteins, and cell structures. Vitamin E can help lower the risk of chronic diseases and decrease the aging process by scavenging free radicals.

Immune System Support: Vitamin E improves the performance of immune cells, supporting a strong immune system. It aids the body's defense mechanisms against diseases and infections.

Skin Health: Due to its ability to support healthy skin, vitamin E is frequently used in skincare products and dietary supplements. It encourages skin hydration, lessens skin inflammation, and could offer UV radiation damage protection. Vitamin E is also applied topically by some people to treat skin issues like scars and wrinkles.

Cardiovascular Health: Vitamin E may be beneficial for cardiovascular health. It may be able to aid in preventing the oxidation of LDL cholesterol, also known as "bad" cholesterol, which is a crucial stage in the emergence of cardiovascular illnesses. To completely comprehend its implications on heart health, more study is necessary.

Eye Health: Age-related macular degeneration (AMD) and cataracts, two prevalent eye disorders that can cause vision loss, may be prevented by vitamin E.

Brain Health: According to some research, vitamin E may help maintain cognitive function and lower the risk of cognitive decline in elderly people.

Red Blood Cell Formation: Vitamin E aids in red blood cell health maintenance. Red blood cells transport oxygen throughout the body.

Reproductive Health: Vitamin E contributes to men's regular sperm production and function in the reproductive system. It might aid women in avoiding problems with their pregnancies.

Inflammatory Conditions: Vitamin E may assist the body's own inflammation be reduced, which is advantageous for ailments including rheumatoid arthritis and asthma.

Muscle Health: Vitamin E is crucial for the maintenance of muscle cells and may help prevent muscular damage caused by strenuous exercise.

Anticancer Capabilities: According to some research, vitamin E's antioxidant capabilities may help to prevent some types of cancer. However, the evidence is conflicting, and more study is required.

Vitamin K:

Blood Clotting: Vitamin K's role in the blood clotting process is one of its main activities. The production of numerous proteins involved in the development of clots depends on it. Blood coagulation would be compromised without enough vitamin K, resulting in excessive bleeding and hemorrhage.

Bone Health: Vitamin K, in particular vitamin K2, affects bone health by controlling the calcium that is deposited in bones and teeth. It aids in the activation of the osteocalcin protein, which binds calcium to the bone matrix to strengthen and lessen the likelihood of fractured bones.

Cardiovascular Health: According to recent studies, vitamin K2 may support cardiovascular health by avoiding artery calcification. This might lower the chance of developing heart disease.

Osteoporosis Prevention: Getting enough vitamin K may help prevent the disease and lower the risk of fractures, particularly in postmenopausal women.

Brain Health: Although more research is required to completely understand vitamin K's impact in this respect, it is thought to support brain health.

Skin Health: Vitamin K may aid in reducing skin pigmentation and promoting wound healing; hence several skincare products contain it.

Antioxidant Properties: Mild antioxidant qualities conferred by vitamin K allow it to aid in preventing oxidative cell damage.

Neonatal Health: To prevent a rare bleeding ailment called hemorrhagic disease of the newborn (HDN), newborns are frequently given a vitamin K injection shortly after birth. Because babies have lower quantities of vitamin K and fewer gut microbes to manufacture it, this disease can develop.

Cancer Prevention: Although more research is required in this area, several studies have suggested that adequate vitamin K intake may be linked to a decreased risk of some malignancies.

Vitamin K1:

Blood Clotting: The primary role of vitamin K1 is to promote coagulation and blood clotting. Prothrombin and factors VII, IX, and X are only a few of the proteins in the blood-clotting cascade that need it to be synthesized. When a blood vessel is ruptured, these proteins are essential for the creation of blood clots that stop the bleeding.

Wound Healing: Blood clot development at the site of damage is promoted by vitamin K1, which aids in the body's capacity to mend wounds. This enables the body to heal injured tissue and lessens excessive bleeding.

Prevention of Hemorrhage in Newborns: Newborns are born with low quantities of vitamin K1 and few gut bacteria that can synthesis it, which makes it difficult for them to prevent hemorrhaging. Infants are generally given a vitamin K1 injection soon after delivery to prevent hemorrhagic disease of the newborn (HDN), a rare bleeding disorder.

Maintaining Bone Health: Osteocalcin, a protein that binds calcium to the bone matrix, is activated by vitamin K1, which helps to maintain bone health. Vitamin K2 is more intimately linked to bone health and calcium metabolism, although vitamin K1 also contributes to bone health maintenance.

Cardiovascular Health: According to recent study, vitamin K1 may contribute to cardiovascular health by lowering the risk of artery calcification. Although more research is required in this area, this may help reduce the risk of heart disease.

Antioxidant Properties: Vitamin K1 has a little amount of antioxidant qualities, which implies they may help shield cells from oxidative harm.

Cancer Prevention: Although more research is required in this area, several studies have suggested that adequate vitamin K1 intake may be linked to a decreased risk of some malignancies.

Allicin:

Antimicrobial Properties: Allicin has antibacterial properties, which means it can stop the growth of or actually kill germs including bacteria, fungi, and viruses. Although the degree of its efficiency can vary, it might aid in the treatment of infections.

Antioxidant Activity: Allicin possesses antioxidant qualities, which can help shield cells from the oxidative damage brought on by free radicals. Its capacity to lower the risk of chronic diseases may be influenced by this.

Cardiovascular Health: According to certain research, eating garlic and allicin may be good for your heart. Allicin may help enhance blood vessel health, lower cholesterol, and lower blood pressure. The risk of heart disease may be decreased as a result of these factors.

Effects on Inflammation: Allicin might be anti-inflammatory, which could help lessen inflammation in the body. Since chronic inflammation is linked to a number of disorders, this effect might be advantageous for general health.

Immune System Support: Allicin may strengthen the immune system by boosting immune cell activity and maybe assisting the body in warding off infections. Allicin may have anticancer characteristics, according to some research, but additional research is required to completely understand how it affects cancer prevention and treatment.

Antioxidant Support for the Liver: Allicin may offer the liver antioxidant assistance. The liver is important for detoxification.

Calcium:

Bone Health: The body stores around 99% of its calcium in the bones and teeth, where it supports the bones' structural integrity and aids in maintaining bone density. In order to prevent osteoporosis and lower the risk of fractures, it is crucial to consume enough calcium throughout life, along with other minerals like vitamin D.

Muscle Contraction: Calcium is a key component in the contraction of muscles. A nerve signal that reaches a muscle causes calcium ions that are stored there to be released. When these calcium ions interact with proteins, muscle fibers can contract.

Nerve Function: Calcium is important for the transmission of nerve signals in the nervous system. Neurotransmitters are chemical messengers that transfer impulses between nerve cells, and it aids in controlling their release.

Blood Clotting: Calcium is a component of the blood clotting process. When a blood artery is injured, it aids in the activation of many proteins that are involved in the formation of blood clots to halt the bleeding.

Cell Signaling: Calcium operates as a secondary messenger in numerous cellular processes, assisting in the control of a number of activities including cell division, the production of hormones and enzymes, and cell growth and differentiation.

Hormone Secretion: The release of various hormones, including insulin, which controls blood sugar levels, and parathyroid hormone (PTH), which aids in controlling calcium levels in the blood, requires calcium.

Blood Pressure Regulation: Calcium affects how tightly and loosely blood vessel walls contract and relax, which helps to control blood pressure.

Enzyme Activation: Calcium functions as a cofactor for several enzymes involved in procedures like digestion, energy metabolism, and DNA synthesis. This process is known as enzyme activation.

Maintenance of pH Balance: The body's acid-base balance must be maintained for normal physiological function, and calcium ions assist in this process.

Cell Adhesion: Calcium plays a part in cell adhesion, assisting cells to adhere to one another to build tissues and organs.

Choline:

Cell Membrane Structure: Choline is a part of phospholipids, which are crucial elements of the structural makeup of cell membranes. For cells to function and communicate, the integrity and fluidity of their membranes must be preserved.

Neurotransmitter Synthesis: Choline is a precursor for the neurotransmitter acetylcholine, which is essential for memory, muscular control, and nerve function. Normal cognitive function is supported by an adequate choline intake.

Liver Health: Choline plays a role in the transportation and metabolism of fats in the liver, which affects liver health. It aids in preventing the buildup of fat in the liver, which is crucial for the health of the liver. Fatty liver disease can result from choline shortage.

Cell Signaling: The manufacture of certain signaling molecules and second messengers in the body depends on choline, which is involved in a number of cells signaling processes.

DNA Synthesis: Choline is required to produce DNA and is also important for cell development and division.

Brain Development: Normal brain growth depends on getting enough choline during pregnancy and early childhood. On children's memory and cognitive function, it might have a permanent effect.

Methyl Group Donor: Choline is a methyl donor, which indicates that it can give methyl groups to different compounds. This is crucial for a number of biochemical procedures, such as the control of gene expression, detoxification, and homocysteine metabolism.

Immunity and Inflammation: By affecting the creation of specific immune cells and molecules, choline may have anti-inflammatory effects and assist the immune system.

Heart Health: According to some research, choline intake may be connected to a lower risk of developing heart disease because it helps control homocysteine levels, which are linked to heart health.

Choline Deficiency and Disease Prevention: Preventing diseases associated with choline insufficiency, such as fatty liver disease, muscular damage, and neurological issues, can be done by ensuring adequate choline intake.

Curcumin:

Anti-Inflammatory Properties: Curcumin is a powerful natural substance with anti-inflammatory properties. By preventing the function of inflammatory chemicals and enzymes, it can aid in the reduction of inflammatory processes in the body. Since chronic inflammation is connected to many chronic diseases, curcumin's anti-inflammatory properties may have a variety of positive health impacts.

Antioxidant Activity: Curcumin has antioxidant properties, which means it can fight off dangerous free radicals that can harm DNA and cells. Its antioxidant qualities assist in defending cells against oxidative stress and lower the risk of chronic illnesses linked to oxidative damage.

Pain Relief: Curcumin may have analgesic (pain-relieving) effects, according to some research. It might be useful in treating pain brought on by illnesses like arthritis and tight muscles.

Supports Joint Health: Curcumin's anti-inflammatory and antioxidant characteristics may be able to help lessen the signs and symptoms of rheumatoid arthritis and osteoarthritis. Through cartilage protection, it might help promote joint health.

Digestive Health: Curcumin may improve digestion by encouraging the formation of bile, which facilitates it, and by easing indigestion and bloating symptoms. Additionally, it might protect the digestive system.

Heart Health: According to certain studies, curcumin may be beneficial for heart health. By lowering risk factors like oxidative stress and inflammation, it might assist to enhance cardiovascular function.

Brain Function: Curcumin may improve cognitive function and brain health. The growth factor known as brain-derived neurotrophic factor (BDNF), which is important for brain health and the development of new synaptic connections, may be supported by this substance.

Cancer Prevention: Several studies indicate that curcumin may have anti-cancer properties, while more research is required in this area. It might stop cancer cells from multiplying, stop tumors from spreading, and boost the effects of chemotherapy.

Antibacterial and Antiviral Properties: Curcumin possesses antibacterial and antiviral characteristics that have been shown in some research, which may aid the body in warding off infections.

Skin Health: Curcumin topical use may be advantageous for skin health. It might facilitate wound healing, lessen the visibility of scars, and ease some skin disorders.

Iron:

Oxygen Transport: One of iron's main jobs is to make it easier for oxygen to go from the lungs to the body's cells. Hemoglobin, a protein present in red blood cells, needs iron to function properly. In the lungs, hemoglobin binds to oxygen, transports it through the bloodstream, and releases it in the cells where it is used to produce energy.

Energy Production: Iron participates in the electron transport chain, a sequence of chemical events that take place inside mitochondria, which are the cell's energy-producing organelles. The creation of adenosine triphosphate (ATP), the main source of energy for cells, depends on this chain.

Immune Function: Iron supports the immune system and aids in immunological function. It is essential for immune cells to function properly and aids the body's defense against diseases and infections.

Cognitive Function: Iron is crucial for appropriate brain development and cognitive function, especially in newborns and young children. Cognitive problems might result from an iron deficit during key developmental stages.

Detoxification: Iron participates in the liver's detoxification process, where it aids in the metabolization and removal of potentially toxic compounds from the body.

DNA Synthesis: Iron is necessary for the creation of DNA, the genetic material found in all cells. It is essential for cell development and division.

Collagen Synthesis: Collagen is a structural protein that maintains the skin, blood vessels, tendons, and bones. Iron is involved in collagen synthesis.

Hormone Production: Iron is required for the synthesis of several hormones, including those that affect growth and sexual development.

Red Blood Cell Formation: Iron is necessary for the creation of new red blood cells, which is a process called hemoglobin synthesis. Anemia, which is characterized by a lower level of red blood cells and a diminished ability to deliver oxygen, can result from an iron deficit.

Heart Health: Adequate iron levels are crucial for heart health since low iron levels can raise the risk of heart disease and cause heart palpitations associated with anemia.

Magnesium:

Energy Production: Magnesium is a cofactor in a number of enzymatic processes that contribute to the production of energy. By promoting the synthesis of adenosine triphosphate (ATP), the main source of energy for cells, it aids in the conversion of food into energy.

Muscle Function: Magnesium is essential for the contraction and relaxation of muscles. It is important for muscle fibers to operate properly, especially the heart muscle. Magnesium levels that are adequate support normal muscular tone and guard against cramping.

Nervous System Function: Magnesium aids in the transmission of nerve signals in the nervous system. It contributes to appropriate nerve function and coordination by controlling the activity of neurotransmitters and neuromuscular junctions.

Bone Health: Magnesium is an essential part of bone structure and promotes bone health. It aids in controlling the metabolism of calcium and vitamin D, both of which are necessary for bone mineralization. Osteoporosis risk may be lowered by consuming enough magnesium.

Heart Health: Magnesium has a crucial role in sustaining heart health. It improves blood vessel health, controls heart rhythm, and can help lower blood pressure. Lack of magnesium is linked to a higher risk of cardiovascular disorders.

Blood Sugar Control: Magnesium aids in the relaxation of blood vessels, which may help with blood pressure regulation. It can aid in lowering blood pressure and preventing hypertension.

Blood Pressure Regulation: Magnesium helps relax blood vessels and may contribute to the regulation of blood pressure. It can help prevent hypertension (high blood pressure).

DNA and RNA Synthesis: Magnesium is required for the stability and production of DNA and RNA, the genetic material in cells. It contributes to cell development and division.

Antioxidant Activity: Magnesium contains antioxidant qualities that can help shield cells from the oxidative damage brought on by free radicals.

Protein Synthesis: Magnesium is necessary for the body to produce proteins during protein synthesis. It plays a role in the enzymes that help with protein synthesis being activated.

Detoxification: Magnesium aids in the metabolization and removal of toxins from the body in the liver during the detoxification process.

Mood and Mental Health: Magnesium may have a calming effect on the nervous system and can help lessen the feelings of anxiety and sadness, according to research on mood and mental health. Additionally, it might aid cognitive function.

Digestive Health: Magnesium can aid in the relaxation of the muscles of the digestive tract, which promotes regular bowel movements and averts constipation.

Manganese:

Antioxidant Activity: Manganese has antioxidant properties and is a cofactor for the antioxidant enzyme superoxide dismutase (SOD). These enzymes aid in preventing oxidative cell damage brought on by free radicals, which can speed up aging and the onset of many diseases.

Bone Health: Manganese is necessary for the growth and upkeep of strong bones. It contributes to the production of proteoglycans, which are crucial parts of connective tissues, such as bone cartilage. Bone structure and function are supported by a sufficient manganese intake.

Cartilage Formation: The formation of glycosaminoglycans (GAGs), which are substances found in cartilage and other connective tissues, requires manganese. GAGs support the flexibility and health of joints.

Wound Healing: Manganese plays a role in the process of healing wounds. Collagen, a structural protein that aids in tissue repair, is formed as a result of it.

Metabolism: Enzymes involved in metabolism, such as those that aid in the breakdown of amino acids, cholesterol, and carbohydrates, require manganese as a cofactor. Additionally, it contributes to the synthesis of fatty acids and the metabolism of glucose.

Neurotransmitter Regulation: The chemical messengers known as neurotransmitters, which are used to carry messages between nerve cells, are regulated by manganese. It helps to make and keep neurotransmitters like serotonin and norepinephrine in good working order.

Reproductive Health: Manganese is necessary for the formation of healthy sperm and is vital for reproductive health. It contributes to the production of sex hormones and might aid in normal reproductive function.

Blood Sugar Regulation: Blood Sugar Control: According to some research, manganese may aid in blood sugar control by affecting insulin release and glucose metabolism. More study is, however, required in this field.

Immune System: Manganese is necessary for the immune system to operate normally. It supports immunological responses to infections and aids in the activation of some immune cells.

Detoxification: Manganese participates in the liver's detoxification processes, where it aids in the body's metabolization and removal of pollutants.

Molybdenum:

Cofactor for Enzymes: Molybdenum serves as a cofactor for a number of enzymes in the body. Its role as a cofactor for the enzyme's sulfite oxidase, aldehyde oxidase, and xanthine oxidase is most notable. These enzymes take part in crucial metabolic processes.

Purine Metabolism: The nitrogen-containing substances known as purines, which are contained in DNA and RNA, are metabolized by molybdenum. For instance, xanthine oxidase turns purines like xanthine and hypoxanthine into uric acid, which is then eliminated through the urine. Gout is one of the disorders that can result from purine metabolism dysregulation.

Sulfite detoxification: Sulfite oxidase, an enzyme that detoxifies sulfites in the body, requires molybdenum to function. Sulfites are food preservatives that can be created as byproducts of the metabolism of amino acids that include sulfur. Sulfites are changed into less harmful and excretable sulfates by the enzyme sulfite oxidase.

Detoxification of Aldehydes: Aldehyde oxidase, another molybdenum-dependent enzyme, plays a role in the metabolism of various aldehydes, which are chemical substances that can be present in some meals and are created during the metabolism of alcohol. These substances are detoxified by aldehyde oxidase.

Nitrogen Metabolism: By taking part in reactions that transform amino acids into other substances, molybdenum indirectly contributes to nitrogen metabolism. It aids in the transformation of sulfur-containing metabolites formed from amino acids like cysteine and methionine.

Enzyme Activation: Molybdenum serves as a cofactor for other enzymes that are involved in the body's creation of different compounds and the metabolism of energy.

Phosphorus:

Bone and Teeth Health: The majority of the body's phosphorus is found in the bones and teeth, where it mixes with calcium to provide them strength and rigidity. For bone tissue to form, remain healthy, and be repaired, phosphorus is necessary.

Cellular Energy Production: Adenosine triphosphate (ATP), the main molecule that stores and distributes energy within cells, is made up in large part of phosphorus. The structure and operation of ATP, also known as the "energy currency" of the cell, are both dependent on phosphorus.

DNA and RNA Synthesis: Phosphorus is a component of DNA and RNA, the genetic components that make up a cell. It is crucial to the synthesis, replication, and repair of DNA and RNA.

Cellular Signaling: Phosphorus has a role in cellular signaling pathways, assisting in the transmission of messages both within and between cells. In order to add phosphate groups to proteins, a process known as phosphorylation is frequently used in cellular control.

Acid-Base Balance: Phosphorus contributes to the maintenance of the body's acid-base balance by assisting in the control of the pH of biological fluids. It functions as a buffer, assisting in preventing abrupt pH shifts.

Muscle Function: Phosphorus is necessary for both muscle contraction and relaxation. Calcium ions, which are essential for muscular activity, are released and used by it.

Nerve Function: Phosphorus plays a part in the transmission of nerve signals and nerve activity. It plays a role in how action potentials in nerve cells are produced and spread.

Kidney Function: Blood phosphorus levels are closely regulated by the kidneys, which perform the function of the kidneys. By eliminating extra phosphorus, the kidneys aid in keeping the body's pH levels in check.

Metabolism: Phosphorus has a role in a number of metabolic activities, including the metabolism of proteins, lipids, and carbohydrates. It functions as a cofactor for numerous enzymes involved in these metabolic pathways.

Cell Membrane Structure: Phosphorus plays a significant role in the structure of cell membranes, where it interacts with lipids to produce phospholipids. Cell membrane integrity and structure are preserved by phospholipids.

Respiratory Function: Phosphorus aids in the blood's ability to transport oxygen during respiration. It is a component of a substance called 2,3-diphosphoglycerate (2,3-DPG), which has an impact on how hemoglobin in red blood cells binds to and releases oxygen.

Piperine:

Enhancement of Nutrient Absorption: Piperine's capacity to improve the absorption of numerous nutrients from the digestive tract is one of its most well-known functions. It accomplishes this by blocking specific gastrointestinal enzymes, particularly those involved in the metabolism and excretion of many medicines and nutrients, such as cytochrome P450 and UDP-glucuronosyltransferase.

Piperine can boost the bioavailability of compounds like curcumin (found in turmeric), resveratrol (found in red wine), and specific vitamins and minerals by blocking these enzymes.

Effects on Inflammation: Piperine might reduce inflammation. The anti-inflammatory properties of piperine may aid in lowering inflammation and the related health concerns as inflammation is a major contributing factor in many chronic diseases.

Antioxidant Activity: Piperine has antioxidant qualities, which means it can aid in scavenging dangerous free radicals and lowering oxidative stress in the body. Its possible health advantages may be a result of this antioxidant action.

Potential Weight Management Support: Potential Support for Weight Management: Research suggests that piperine may help people manage their weight. It might aid in enhancing metabolism and reducing fat cell development. Additionally, piperine may indirectly enhance overall health, which is vital for weight management, by improving nutrient absorption.

Digestive Health: By encouraging the pancreatic release of digestive enzymes and enhancing gastrointestinal motility, piperine may enhance digestive health. This might help with vitamin absorption and meal digestion.

Mood and Cognitive Function: Some research points to piperine's potential for improving mood and cognitive performance. It might affect brain neurotransmitter activity and promote mental health.

Pain Relief: Piperine's possible analgesic (pain-relieving) properties have been researched. By altering pain signaling pathways, it may assist in reducing discomfort and pain.

Effects of Thermogenesis: Piperine may have qualities that cause a rise in body temperature and metabolic rate. Its potential involvement in weight management may be influenced by this impact.

Potential Anti-Cancer Effects: Some studies have looked into the anti-cancer effects of piperine. Certain cancer cells' ability to grow and spread may be hampered. More study is, however, required in this field.

Antibacterial and Antifungal Activity: Piperine has been shown to have antibacterial and antifungal qualities. It might aid in preventing the development of dangerous germs and fungi inside the body.

Potassium:

Electrolyte Balance: Potassium, along with sodium and chloride, is one of the body's major electrolytes. The fluid equilibrium within and around cells, tissues, and organs is preserved by these electrolytes. Maintaining optimal cell activity and general hydration depends on this equilibrium.

Nerve Function: Potassium is necessary for the proper operation of the nervous system and the signaling of the nervous system. Action potentials, electrical signals that move along nerve cells to relay information across the nervous system, are produced with its assistance.

Muscle Function: Potassium is essential for the proper operation of muscles, including skeletal muscles (muscles you can control, such as those in your arms and legs) and smooth muscles (muscles that regulate blood vessels and involuntary activities). Potassium aids in controlling muscular relaxation and contraction.

Heart Health: Potassium is essential for sustaining a healthy heart's rhythm and function. It aids in controlling the electrical impulses responsible for heart contraction regulation. A lower risk of heart arrhythmias and hypertension (high blood pressure) is linked to adequate potassium intake.

Blood Pressure Control: By blocking the effects of sodium, potassium helps control blood pressure. A potassium-rich diet can lower blood pressure by encouraging vasodilation (blood vessel relaxation) and lowering the risk of hypertension.

Fluid Balance: Potassium and sodium work together to control the body's fluid balance. The preservation of blood volume, blood pressure, and general hydration depend on this equilibrium.

Kidney Function: Potassium regulates the reabsorption and excretion of different chemicals, including sodium, potassium, and water, which helps to support renal function. The kidneys support appropriate blood potassium levels.

Acid-Base Balance: By regulating the pH of biological fluids, potassium helps to maintain the body's acid-base balance.

Metabolism: Several metabolic processes, such as the transformation of glucose (blood sugar) into glycogen (stored energy) and the production of proteins and nucleic acids, need potassium.

Bone Health: Calcium and phosphorus are more closely linked to bone health, but potassium also plays a role in maintaining a healthy acid-base balance, which may aid to prevent calcium loss from bones.

Quercetin:

Antioxidant Activity: Quercetin's high antioxidant properties allow it to effectively combat the body's dangerous free radicals. This antioxidant action aids in preventing oxidative cell damage, which is linked to a number of chronic illnesses and aging.

Anti-Inflammatory Properties: Quercetin has anti-inflammatory properties that may aid in reducing inflammation in the body. Numerous medical disorders, including heart disease and arthritis, are associated with chronic inflammation.

Support for the Immune System: Quercetin may have immune-modulating qualities. Its ability to increase the activity of immune cells like macrophages and lymphocytes, which are essential in defending the body against infections, has been explored.

Heart Health: According to certain studies, quercetin may offer advantages for the heart. By promoting vascular health and lowering oxidative stress, it may help to enhance blood vessel function, lower blood pressure, and minimize the risk of heart disease.

Allergy Relief: Quercetin has been researched for its ability to lessen allergy symptoms like sneezing, runny noses, and itchy eyes. It may have anti-allergic characteristics. Mast cells, which release histamines during allergic reactions, may benefit from its stabilization.

Respiratory Health: Quercetin has been investigated for its ability to promote respiratory health. It may lessen symptoms like coughing and congestion and lessen the severity of respiratory infections like the common cold and the flu.

Exercise Performance: According to some research, quercetin may increase exercise endurance while lowering inflammation and oxidative stress brought on by exercise. Athletes and anyone who engages in demanding physical activity might benefit from it.

Cognitive Function: Quercetin may help to support the health of the brain and cognitive function. Its potential to safeguard neurons and enhance learning and memory has been studied.

Skin Health: Quercetin's anti-inflammatory and antioxidant capabilities may help control skin disorders like eczema and psoriasis as well as protect against the damaging effects of UV radiation.

Blood Sugar Control: According to some research, quercetin may enhance insulin sensitivity and help regulate blood sugar levels, which may be helpful for people with diabetes or at risk of acquiring the disease.

Selenium:

Antioxidant Activity: Selenium has antioxidant properties and functions as a cofactor for some antioxidant enzymes, including glutathione peroxidases. By scavenging damaging free radicals and reactive oxygen species (ROS), these enzymes assist in preventing oxidative damage to cells. The antioxidant capabilities of selenium help lower the risk of chronic conditions like cancer and cardiovascular disease that are brought on by oxidative stress.

Immune System Support: Support for the Immune System: Selenium helps the immune system work properly. It is essential for immune cells to function properly and for the creation of cytokines, which are signaling molecules that control immunological reactions. A sufficient intake of selenium supports the body's fight against illnesses and infections.

Thyroid Function: The conversion of thyroid hormones from their inactive form (thyroxine, or T4) to their active form (triiodothyronine, or T3) depends on selenium. The thyroid gland's healthy operation and the control of metabolism depend on this conversion.

DNA Repair: Selenium has a role in the processes involved in DNA repair. It supports the repair of DNA lesions brought on by numerous sources, including UV radiation and toxins, and aids in the prevention of harm to genetic material.

Cancer Prevention: Selenium may play a part in the prevention of cancer, according to some research. Selenium is believed to have anti-cancer effects in part because of its antioxidant characteristics and capacity to help DNA repair. Selenium and cancer risk, however, have a complicated association that can change depending on a variety of conditions.

Heart Health: Selenium may be beneficial for cardiovascular health. It aids in lowering oxidative stress and inflammation, both of which are risk factors for heart disease. According to several studies, getting enough selenium may lower your chance of developing coronary heart disease.

Male Reproductive Health: Selenium is crucial for the health of the male reproductive system. It is essential for both sperm motility and production. Men who are selenium deficient may experience problems getting pregnant.

Brain Health: Selenium may help to support cognitive function and lower the risk of neurodegenerative illnesses, which is good news for people with brain health. It might lessen the risk of oxidative damage to neurons.

Anti-Inflammatory Effects: Selenium has anti-inflammatory actions that may help lower the chance of developing chronic inflammatory disorders. These effects are a result of the antioxidant qualities that it possesses.

Hair and Skin Health: Selenium has a role in maintaining healthy Hair and Skin. It promotes the health of hair follicles and skin cells.

Zinc:

Immune System Support: Zinc is well-known for playing a crucial part in the healthy operation of the immune system. It aids in regulating the generation and function of immune cells that are essential for protecting the body against infections, such as T lymphocytes and white blood cells.

Wound Healing: Zinc plays a role in several stages of the healing process for wounds. It is crucial for the healing of cuts, burns, and other wounds because it encourages cell development and tissue restoration.

DNA Synthesis and Repair: Zinc is necessary for the synthesis, replication, and repair of DNA. It is essential for preserving the stability and integrity of the genetic material.

Enzyme Function: Zinc is a cofactor needed by numerous body enzymes to catalyze biological reactions. These enzymes are essential for functions like digestion, energy metabolism, and chemical synthesis.

Antioxidant Defense: Zinc has antioxidant capabilities that help shield cells from the oxidative damage brought on by free radicals. Together with other antioxidants like vitamin C and vitamin E, it effectively combats dangerous free radicals.

Taste and Smell Perception: Zinc is necessary for taste and smell receptors to operate normally. Alterations in taste perception and a decreased capacity to perceive scents can result from a zinc shortage.

Hormone Regulation: Zinc contributes to the control of hormones and aids the endocrine system's operation. It contributes to the synthesis and function of numerous hormones, including thyroid and insulin.

Growth and Development: During childhood, adolescence, and pregnancy, zinc is essential for healthy growth and development. It is essential for the production of proteins as well as the growth of tissues and organs.

Skin Health: Zinc promotes healthy skin and can help treat diseases like eczema and acne. It encourages skin cells to operate normally and might have anti-inflammatory properties.

Eye Health: Zinc is crucial for sustaining eyesight and is present in high amounts in the retina of the eye. It is especially crucial for the macula, a region of the retina that controls central vision.

Bone Health: Zinc has a role in the mineralization and development of bones. It aids in the formation and preservation of strong bones.

Mental health: Some research has revealed a connection between zinc deficiency and mental health conditions like anxiety and depression. Neurotransmitter modulation and mood stabilization may be aided by zinc.

Amino Acid Benefits

Arginine:

Nitric Oxide Synthesis: Nitric oxide (NO), a molecule that acts as a vasodilator, is produced from the amino acid arginine. Blood vessels are relaxed by NO, which improves circulation and blood flow. The control of blood pressure and cardiovascular health depend on this function.

Wound Healing and Tissue Repair: Tissue repair and wound healing depend on the production of collagen and other proteins, both of which are facilitated by arginine. It aids in the growth of fresh blood vessels where there have been wounds.

Immune Function: Arginine supports the generation and functioning of immune cells, contributing to the health of the immune system. Both innate and adaptive immune responses involve it.

Hormone Regulation: Arginine plays a role in the release of growth hormone (GH) from the pituitary gland, which regulates hormones. It can encourage the release of GH, which is crucial for promoting muscular growth.

Detoxification: Ammonia, a waste product of protein breakdown, is removed from the body by arginine. For people with liver illness or other disorders that impact ammonia metabolism, this is especially crucial.

Kidney Function: Arginine is essential for maintaining healthy kidney function and, under some circumstances, may help guard against kidney injury.

Cognitive Health: According to some research, arginine may aid in memory and cognitive function. It contributes to the production of neurotransmitters and controls cerebral blood flow.

Sperm Production and Fertility: Sperm production and male fertility are supported by arginine, which also contributes to sperm production. It contributes to sperm production and the preservation of normal sperm function.

Collagen Production: The formation of collagen, a structural protein present in skin, cartilage, and connective tissues, requires arginine. It helps wounds heal and maintain healthy skin.

Antioxidant Properties: Arginine has antioxidant properties and can help protect cells from oxidative damage caused by free radicals.

Cysteine:

Disulfide Bond Formation: Cysteine has a thiol (-SH) group in its side chain, which can join with other cysteine molecules to form powerful chemical bonds known as disulfide bonds (-S-S-). Many enzymes, antibodies, and structural proteins like keratin in hair and nails depend on disulfide bonds for their structure and stability.

Antioxidant Activity: Cysteine is a precursor of the tripeptide glutathione, one of the body's most potent antioxidants, which has antioxidant properties. Glutathione aids in the elimination of negative free radicals and shields cells from oxidative stress. By attaching to and assisting in the elimination of heavy metals and poisons from the body, it also contributes to the detoxification process.

Immune System Support: Cysteine is essential for the immune system to function properly. The body's defense against infections depends on the generation of antibodies, which is one of its functions.

Respiratory Health: N-acetylcysteine (NAC), a mucolytic agent, has cysteine as one of its ingredients. In diseases like cystic fibrosis and chronic obstructive pulmonary disease (COPD), NAC is used therapeutically to help thin and loosen mucus in the respiratory system, making it simpler to clear and improve breathing.

Detoxification: Glutathione production is only one aspect of cysteine's role in detoxification. It is a part of the detoxification process for a number of substances, including narcotics, toxins, and contaminants.

Hair and Skin Health: Cysteine helps produce keratin, a structural protein that is present in the Hair, Skin, and Nails. For the tissues to remain healthy and attractive, it is crucial.

Collagen Production: The formation of collagen, a structural protein present in connective tissues, bones, and blood vessels, requires cysteine. For these tissues to remain strong and intact, collagen is essential.

Metabolism: Homocysteine, an amino acid linked to cardiovascular health, is metabolized with the help of cysteine. It is transformed into cystathionine, which undergoes additional metabolism to produce healthy substances like cysteine and taurine.

Neurotransmitter Production: Cysteine has a role in the synthesis of a number of neurotransmitters, including serotonin and dopamine. These neurotransmitters are crucial for maintaining cognitive function and controlling mood.

Glycine:

Neurotransmitter: Glycine is a neurotransmitter that acts as an inhibitor in the central nervous system. It functions as a natural relaxant by soothing the brain and spinal cord. The nervous system's glycine receptors are involved in controlling how muscles contract and move.

Collagen Production: Glycine is a crucial part of the structural protein collagen, which helps to build the connective tissues in the body, such as the skin, tendons, ligaments, and cartilage. For these tissues to remain strong and intact, collagen is crucial.

Protein Synthesis: Glycine functions as an amino acid in the production of proteins. It is one of the 20 amino acids that the body uses to construct proteins.

Detoxification: Glycine is crucial for the liver's ability to effectively detoxify a variety of chemicals. It has a role in the production of glutathione, a potent antioxidant that fights free radicals and toxic chemicals. Additionally, glycine is important for the conjugation of poisons for excretion.

Creatine Synthesis: Glycine is one of the precursors utilized in the synthesis of creatine, a substance that gives muscles energy during brief bursts of vigorous exercise.

Metabolism: Glycine participates in a number of metabolic processes, including the transformation of serine into glycine, which is necessary for the creation of DNA and RNA as well as other significant molecules.

Wound Healing: Glycine is crucial for both tissue repair and wound healing. It stimulates the regeneration of injured tissues and aids in the creation of collagen.

Gastrointestinal Health: Glycine helps to keep the digestive system in good condition. Bile salts are produced as a result of its involvement, and these salts help in fat digestion and absorption.

Immune System Support: Glycine plays a crucial role in the creation of antibodies, which are crucial elements of the immune system's fight against pathogens.

Anti-Inflammatory Properties: Glycine may contain anti-inflammatory effects, which could assist to lessen inflammation in the body, according to some research.

Cognitive Function: Glycine may play a part in memory and cognitive function. It is involved in the control of brain-function-critical neurotransmitters including glutamate and glycine.

Histidine:

Precursor to Histamine: Histidine, a chemical involved in immunological responses, allergic reactions, and the control of stomach acid, is a precursor of histamine. In reaction to damage, illness, or allergies, immune cells and mast cells produce histamine.

Protein Synthesis: Histidine plays a crucial role in the production of proteins. It contributes to the biological activities of several proteins, enzymes, and peptides by being incorporated into their structures.

Metal Binding: Histidine is a metal ion ligand, especially for transition metals including copper, zinc, and iron. It affects the design and operation of metalloproteins.

Neurotransmitter Regulation: Histidine plays an important role in the modulation of neurotransmitters in the brain. It can be changed into the neurotransmitter histamine, which has a role in the processes involved in alertness, arousal, and cognitive function.

Immune System Function: Histidine is crucial for the immune system's ability to react to allergens and pathogens. In response to immunological challenges, it helps to activate immune cells and produce histamine.

Blood pH Regulation: Histidine can function as a buffer to aid in regulating blood pH. To maintain the acid-base balance of the organism, it can receive or release protons (H+ ions).
Histidine is involved in both tissue repair and wound healing. It contributes to the production of collagen, a structural protein vital to the health of connective tissues including skin.

Mucin Synthesis: Histidine plays a role in the synthesis of the glycoprotein known as mucin, which serves as a barrier of defense in the mucous membranes of the gastrointestinal tract and other mucous membranes.

Anti-Inflammatory Properties: Histidine may contain anti-inflammatory qualities that can help moderate inflammatory reactions in the body, according to some research.

Red Blood Cell Formation: Histidine has a role in the production of hemoglobin, the oxygen-carrying protein found in red blood cells. Heme, which includes histidine, is a component of hemoglobin.

Cognitive Function: Histidine's possible contribution to memory and cognitive function is still being investigated. It is thought to contribute to the modulation of neurotransmitters that influence cognitive functions.

Isoleucine:

Protein Synthesis: Isoleucine, like all other amino acids, is necessary for the body's protein synthesis process. It contributes to the biological activities of several proteins, enzymes, and peptides by being incorporated into their structures.

Energy Production: Isoleucine is a branched-chain amino acid (BCAA), along with leucine and valine, that is used in the production of energy. Because they may be digested directly in muscle tissue, BCAAs are exceptional in that they can be used as a source of energy during physical activity or other times when more energy is needed.

Muscle Metabolism: Isoleucine is an essential component of the metabolism and repair of muscles. It aids in the growth and repair of muscle tissue and controls the synthesis of muscle proteins.

Blood Sugar Regulation: Leucine, valine, and isoleucine are all a part of the process that controls blood sugar levels. The pancreas' ability to release insulin can be stimulated by BCAAs, which helps minimize post-meal blood sugar spikes.

Hemoglobin Formation: The formation of hemoglobin, the protein present in red blood cells that delivers oxygen from the lungs to tissues all over the body, involves the amino acid isoleucine. Heme, which includes isoleucine, is a component of hemoglobin.

Immune System Support: Isoleucine is essential for the health of the immune system. It plays a role in immune cell activity and antibody synthesis, which strengthens the body's ability to fight off infections.

Wound Healing: Isoleucine is necessary for both tissue repair and wound healing. Collagen is a structural protein necessary for the health of skin and other connective tissues, and it plays a part in its creation.

Neurotransmitter Regulation: Isoleucine participates in both the synthesis and regulation of neurotransmitters in the brain. These neurotransmitters are crucial for maintaining cognitive function and controlling mood.

Detoxification: Isoleucine has a role in the body's detoxification of substances containing nitrogen.

Leucine:

Protein Synthesis: Leucine is a crucial component of protein synthesis, which is how the body creates and repairs proteins. In particular in muscle tissue, it functions as a signaling molecule to start and accelerate protein synthesis. Leucine is especially significant for athletes and anyone doing weight training since it is essential for muscle growth and repair.

Muscle Health: Leucine, along with isoleucine and valine, is one of the branched-chain amino acids (BCAAs) important for maintaining muscle health. The usefulness of BCAAs to support muscular health is well documented.

Particularly during periods of severe activity or when the body is in a catabolic state (such as during fasting), leucine aids in preventing the breakdown of muscle protein.

Energy Production: Leucine can be used to produce energy during prolonged exercise or times when there is a greater need for it. It can be transformed into glucose in the liver (gluconeogenesis) and used as fuel by many organs.

Blood Sugar Regulation: Leucine, along with isoleucine and valine, is involved in the regulation of blood sugar levels. The pancreas' ability to release insulin can be stimulated by BCAAs, which helps minimize post-meal blood sugar spikes.

Wound Healing: Leucine is necessary for both tissue repair and wound healing. The stability of skin and connective tissues depends on the manufacture of collagen, a structural protein.

Immune System Support: Leucine is essential for the health of the immune system. It plays a role in immune cell activity and antibody synthesis, which strengthens the body's ability to fight off infections.

Neurotransmitter Regulation: The modulation of neurotransmitters in the brain is aided by leucine, which is involved in their production. The regulation of mood and cognitive process are both influenced by these neurotransmitters.

Hormone Regulation: Leucine may affect the hormones growth hormone (GH) and insulin-like growth factor 1 (IGF-1), which are crucial for development of the muscles and overall health, from being released into the body.

Bone Health: Leucine may improve bone health and may help raise bone density, which may help lower the risk of osteoporosis, according to some research.

Lysine:
Protein Synthesis: Lysine is a key protein building block and is necessary for the body's production of many different proteins. The composition and operation of tissues, enzymes, hormones, and other biological substances all depend on proteins.

Collagen Formation: Lysine is essential for the synthesis of collagen, a structural protein that gives skin, cartilage, bones, and other connective tissues their strength and integrity. Joint health, skin health, and wound healing all depend on collagen.

Calcium Absorption: Lysine is a component of the process by which calcium is absorbed from the gastrointestinal system. For the maintenance of sturdy and healthy bones, adequate calcium absorption is necessary.

Enzyme Function: Lysine is a component of enzymes that are involved in a number of metabolic processes. It supports the functioning of these enzymes, which is important for procedures including fatty acid synthesis, glucose metabolism, and energy production.

Immune System Support: Support for the Immune System: Lysine aids the immune system in its operation. It has a role in producing antibodies, which are vital for the body's ability to fight off infections.

Hormone and Enzyme Production: Lysine is involved in the manufacture of a number of hormones and enzymes, including carnitine, which is necessary for the metabolism of fatty acids and the creation of energy.

Wound Healing: Lysine is critical for both tissue repair and wound healing. It stimulates the regeneration of injured tissues and aids in the creation of collagen.

Antiviral Properties: Lysine may have antiviral characteristics, particularly in the setting of herpes simplex virus (HSV) infections, according to certain research. Occasionally, lysine supplements are used to control or stop HSV outbreaks, although more research is required in this area.

Bone Health: Lysine may help to maintain bone health by encouraging the production of collagen and the absorption of calcium.

Methionine:

Protein Synthesis: Methionine is a key component of proteins and is necessary for the body's production of many different proteins. The composition and operation of tissues, enzymes, hormones, and other biological substances all depend on proteins.

Methylation Reactions: Methylation Reactions: S-adenosylmethionine (SAMe), a substance involved in a variety of methylation reactions in the body, is produced from methionine. The crucial biochemical process of methylation is involved in the expression of genes, cell division, detoxification, and the metabolism of hormones and neurotransmitters.

Antioxidant Properties: Methionine has antioxidant properties since it includes sulfur. It aids in defending cells against the oxidative harm brought on by free radicals.

Detoxification: Methionine aids in the detoxification of a number of compounds, including toxic chemicals and heavy metals. It helps create glutathione, a potent antioxidant and detoxifying compound.

Cysteine Synthesis: Methionine is the starting point for the synthesis of cysteine, an additional sulfur-containing amino acid. The production of glutathione and other sulfur-containing molecules requires cysteine.

Lipid Metabolism: Methionine is involved in lipid metabolism, which involves using and breaking down dietary lipids.

Creatine Synthesis: Methionine has a role in the synthesis of creatine, a substance that gives muscles energy during brief bursts of vigorous exercise.

Homocysteine Metabolism: Methionine plays a role in the conversion of homocysteine, an amino acid whose excessive levels are linked to a higher risk of cardiovascular disease. Methionine is involved in the methylation of homocysteine to create cysteine and is also involved in the metabolism of other healthy chemicals.

Wound Healing: Methionine is crucial for the healing of wounds and the repair of tissue. Collagen, a structural protein necessary for the stability of skin and other connective tissues, is synthesized as a result of it.

Phenylalanine:

Protein Synthesis: Phenylalanine is a key protein building ingredient and is required for the production of many different proteins in the body. The composition and operation of tissues, enzymes, hormones, and other biological substances all depend on proteins.

Precursor to Neurotransmitters: Phenylalanine functions as a precursor to a number of significant neurotransmitters in the brain, including:
- Dopamine is a neurotransmitter that is essential for controlling mood, driving motivation, rewarding behavior, and controlling movement.
- Norepinephrine (also known as noradrenaline) is a hormone that affects the body's stress response, alertness, and concentration.
- Epinephrine, often known as adrenaline, causes the "fight-or-flight" reaction, raises heart rate, and primes the body to react swiftly to stress.

Phenylketonuria (PKU) Treatment: Phenylalanine is crucial in the setting of PKU, a hereditary condition that affects the body's capacity to metabolize phenylalanine. In order to prevent the buildup of phenylalanine in the body, which can cause cognitive and neurological problems, people with PKU must adhere to a strict low-phenylalanine diet. In order to deliver necessary amino acids without phenylalanine as part of PKU treatment, phenylalanine-free medical formulations are frequently employed.

Cognitive Function: Phenylalanine and its metabolites, such as dopamine, are involved in memory, attention, and cognitive function. Phenylalanine level variations may have an impact on cognitive functions.

Pain Management: Phenylalanine may be useful in the treatment of pain, according to some studies. It is thought to affect the synthesis of endorphins, which are organic molecules that relieve pain.

Skin and Pigment Formation: Melanin, the pigment that gives skin, hair, and eyes their colors, is produced in part by phenylalanine.

Proline:

Collagen Formation: Proline is essential for the formation of collagen, the most prevalent protein in the human body. Connective tissues like skin, tendons, ligaments, cartilage, and bones all benefit from collagen's ability to provide structure, strength, and flexibility. Proline helps to form the triple-helix structure of collagen molecules, together with amino acids like glycine and lysine.

Wound Healing: Proline is necessary for both tissue repair and wound healing. It contributes to the production of structural proteins like collagen and aids in the repair of damaged tissues.

Joint Health: Collagen contains proline, which is essential for preserving the strength and health of joints. It may improve joint health and mobility by lubricating and cushioning joints.

Heart Health: Proline may play a role in cardiovascular health, according to some research. It contributes to the production of proline-rich proteins that may have an impact on the heart's and blood vessels' functionality.

Immune System Support: Proline is essential for the health of the immune system. It contributes to the immune system's synthesis of antibodies and reactions to wounds and infections.

Antioxidant Properties: Proline contains antioxidant qualities that can help shield cells from the oxidative damage brought on by free radicals. This is especially important for skin health because oxidative stress can speed up aging.

Enzyme and Protein Function: Proline plays a role in the composition and operation of enzymes and proteins. Protein activity and specificity may be impacted by its effects on the three-dimensional shape of proteins.

Collagen-Like Proteins: Proline is also present in proteins other than collagen that have domains that resemble collagen. These proteins are present in a variety of tissues and are involved in structural support, tissue healing, and cell adhesion.

Serine:

Protein Synthesis: Serine is a key protein building ingredient and is required for the production of many different proteins in the body. The composition and operation of tissues, enzymes, hormones, and other biological substances all depend on proteins.

Neurotransmitter Production: Serine is a precursor to a number of crucial neurotransmitters in the brain, such as:
- D-serine: D-serine functions as a neurotransmitter and is important for memory, learning, and synaptic plasticity.
- Glycine is an inhibitory neurotransmitter that affects the sleep-wake cycle, sensory perception, and motor control.

Phospholipid Synthesis: Serine plays a crucial role in the synthesis of phospholipids, which are essential structural elements of cell membranes. The integrity and functionality of cell membranes are maintained by phospholipids.

Creatine Synthesis: Serine has a role in the synthesis of creatine, a substance that gives muscles energy during brief bursts of vigorous exercise.

Immune System Support: Serine is essential for the health of the immunological system. It contributes to the synthesis of antibodies and the immune system's defenses against pathogens.

Detoxification: Serine is involved in the body's process of detoxifying different toxins. It helps create glutathione, a potent antioxidant and detoxifying compound.

Energy Production: Serine can be turned into pyruvate, a crucial intermediary in the metabolism of energy. Pyruvate can be employed in further metabolic processes to create energy or in other metabolic pathways.

Collagen Formation: Serine has a role in the synthesis of collagen, a structural protein that gives connective tissues like skin, tendons, ligaments, and bones their strength and flexibility.

Hemoglobin Synthesis: Serine has a role in the synthesis of hemoglobin, a protein that is found in red blood cells and is responsible for transporting oxygen from the lungs to all of the body's tissues.

Antioxidant Properties: Serine contains antioxidant qualities that can help shield cells from the oxidative damage brought on by free radicals.

Threonine:

Protein Synthesis: Threonine is a crucial component of proteins and is required for the synthesis of a number of different proteins in the body. The composition and operation of tissues, enzymes, hormones, and other biological substances all depend on proteins.

Collagen Formation: Threonine is essential for the synthesis of collagen, a structural protein that gives connective tissues like skin, tendons, ligaments, cartilage, and bones their strength and flexibility. Joint health, skin health, and wound healing all depend on collagen.

Immune System Support: Threonine is essential for the health of the immune system. It contributes to the immune system's synthesis of antibodies and reactions to wounds and infections.

Detoxification: Threonine is involved in the body's process of detoxifying different toxins. It helps create glutathione, a potent antioxidant and detoxifying compound.

Central Nervous System Function: Threonine is a precursor to the amino acid glycine, which is involved in the functioning of the central nervous system. An inhibitory neurotransmitter known as glycine has a sedative impact on the brain.

Enzyme and Protein Function: Function of Enzymes and Proteins: Threonine plays a role in the formation and operation of enzymes and proteins. Protein activity and specificity may be impacted by its effects on the three-dimensional shape of proteins.

Metabolic Pathways: Threonine participates in a number of metabolic processes, including the creation of other amino acids like serine and glycine. It helps maintain the body's general amino acid equilibrium.

Lipid Metabolism: Threonine plays a role in lipid metabolism, which includes the consumption of dietary lipids and the breakdown of those fats.

Brain and Cognitive Health: Research suggests that threonine may have a role in maintaining good brain and cognitive function. It contributes to neurotransmitter production and may have an impact on mood and cognitive function.

Tryptophan:

Precursor to Serotonin: Tryptophan is a precursor to serotonin, a neurotransmitter that is important for regulating mood, emotional stability, and sleep. The neurotransmitter serotonin is frequently referred to as the "feel-good" neurotransmitter due to its impact on mood and emotional stability. Serotonin synthesis requires an adequate intake of tryptophan.

Precursor to Melatonin: Tryptophan serves as a building block for the hormone melatonin, which controls the sleep-wake cycle. Tryptophan levels in the body have an impact on melatonin synthesis. Healthy sleep patterns can be influenced by adequate tryptophan levels.

Protein Synthesis: Tryptophan is a key protein building block and is required for the production of many different proteins in the body. The construction and operation of tissues, enzymes, and hormones depend on proteins.

Niacin (Vitamin B3) Synthesis: Niacin, or vitamin B3, can be produced from tryptophan in the body. Niacin is necessary for a number of biochemical processes, including the metabolism of energy and the preservation of healthy skin, neurons, and digestive organs.

Immune System Support: Tryptophan is important for the health of the immune system. It contributes to the synthesis of antibodies and the immune system's defenses against pathogens.

Regulation of Appetite: According to certain research, tryptophan may have an impact on hunger and food consumption. It might influence how hormones that are connected to appetite are regulated.

Cognition and Memory: Tryptophan is a key player in the cognitive process and memory. It has the potential to impact mood and cognitive functions as a precursor to serotonin.

Stress Response: The body's reaction to stress may be influenced by tryptophan. The neurotransmitter balance that affects stress and anxiety may be impacted.

Valine:

Protein Synthesis: Valine is a key protein building ingredient and is required for the production of many different proteins in the body. The composition and operation of tissues, enzymes, hormones, and other biological substances all depend on proteins.

Energy Production: Valine is one of the branched-chain amino acids (BCAAs), along with leucine and isoleucine, that are used in the production of energy. During physical activity or other times when there is a greater need for energy, BCAAs can be digested directly in muscle tissue and used as a source of fuel.

Muscle Health: Valine, a BCAA, is essential for the metabolism and repair of muscles. It aids in the growth and repair of muscle tissue, works to stop the breakdown of muscle protein, and controls the synthesis of muscle protein.

Blood Sugar Regulation: Valine, along with leucine and isoleucine, is involved in the control of blood sugar levels. The pancreas' ability to release insulin can be stimulated by BCAAs, which helps minimize post-meal blood sugar spikes.

Neurotransmitter Regulation: Valine has the ability to affect how neurotransmitters in the brain are balanced. It challenges tryptophan for brain access, potentially influencing the synthesis of serotonin. The outcome of this competition may affect your mood and cognitive abilities.

Immune System Support: Valine is essential for the health of the immune system. It helps the body fight against infections by assisting in the creation of antibodies and the activation of immune cells.

HMB:

Muscle Preservation and Growth: HMB is frequently marketed as a supplement that can aid in the preservation of muscular tissue and encourage muscle growth. It is thought to function by lessening the breakdown of muscle protein and increasing protein synthesis, which can increase the amount of lean muscle mass, especially while resistance training is taking place.

Strength and Power Improvements: According to some studies, taking HMB supplements may result in gains in strength and power, making them beneficial for athletes and those who engage in strength training or high-intensity workouts. Better performance in sports like weightlifting and sprinting may result from this.

Reduced Muscle Soreness: HMB has been suggested to lessen the soreness brought on by exercise-induced muscle injury. Individuals may be able to recover from strenuous workouts more quickly and perform better in subsequent training sessions as a result.

Improved Exercise Performance: According to some research, HMB can increase aerobic capacity and oxygen use during exercise, which could be advantageous for endurance athletes like runners and cyclists.

Fat Mass Reduction: HMB is primarily linked to benefits for building muscle, although some research indicates that it may also assist in reducing body fat, particularly when paired with exercise. The body composition may improve as a result of this.

Anti-Catabolic Effects: HMB is thought to possess anti-catabolic qualities, which means it might aid in preventing the breakdown of muscle tissue during periods of strenuous exercise or calorie restriction. This is advantageous for people following calorie-restricted diets.

Immune Support: Some research points to HMB's potential to strengthen the immune system, potentially improving general health.

Detoxification: Valine aids in the detoxification of ammonia, a byproduct of the breakdown of proteins. It participates to the urea cycle, which aids in the body's removal of extra ammonia.

Hemoglobin Formation: Valine contributes to the production of hemoglobin, a protein present in red blood cells that transports oxygen from the lungs to tissues all throughout the body.

Wound Healing: Valine is crucial for both tissue repair and wound healing. Collagen, a structural protein necessary for the stability of skin and other connective tissues, is synthesized as a result of it.

Brain Health: Valine and the other BCAAs are thought to contribute to the health and efficiency of the brain. These amino acids may alter mood and mental clarity through influencing the synthesis of neurotransmitters.

Creatine:

ATP Regeneration: Creatine's role in the quick regeneration of adenosine triphosphate (ATP), the main source of energy for cells, is what makes it so well-known. ATP is quickly depleted when you perform short bursts of strong physical activity, like weightlifting or sprinting. Creatine aids in ATP restoration, enabling the continuation of transient, intense efforts.

Muscle Energy: Creatine is stored in the form of creatine phosphate in muscle cells. For a quick supply of energy for muscle contraction during high-intensity exercise, creatine phosphate can transfer its phosphate group to ADP (adenosine diphosphate).

Muscle Growth: Creatine has been demonstrated to increase muscle mass in some people, particularly those who exercise with resistance. It achieves this by promoting protein synthesis and increasing water retention in muscle cells. Over time, this impact may result in increased muscle size and strength.

Exercise Performance: It has been shown that taking a creatine supplement can help you exercise more effectively, especially if you engage in short bursts of high-intensity activity like weightlifting, sprinting, or leaping. It might also lessen the effects of repeated, hard workouts on the muscles.

Brain Health: Recent studies indicate that creatine may have potential advantages for the brain. It may enhance brain health and function by giving brain cells more energy. There has to be more research in these areas, but some studies have looked at the impact of creatine in diseases like Alzheimer's disease and depression.

Neurological Disorders: The use of creatine supplements in the treatment of some neurological disorders, such as some types of muscular dystrophy, has shown promise. In people with these disorders, it can aid in enhancing muscle strength and functionality.

Cardiovascular Health: Some research points to creatine's possible role in enhancing blood vessels and exercise capacity, as well as cardiovascular health. More study is, however, required in this field.

Recovery: By lowering muscle damage and inflammation, creatine may help with post-exercise recovery. Individuals may recover more quickly as a result between challenging sessions.

Summary of Benefits

Benefits from a broth containing these ingredients are antiviral, antioxidant, antimicrobial, anti-inflammatory, anti-cancer, which also supports your eyes, skin, hair, fingernails, muscles, bones, joints, liver, heart, lungs, stomach and brain in addition to being able to help improve your sleep, mood, mental health, reducing depression. It supports your hormones, blood, DNA, growth, reproductive health, digestion, while working synergistically for maximum absorption of the vitamins and nutrients.

There really is a lot to unpack, over and above what I've summarized so at some point, it would be a good idea to go through the complete breakdown of all of the benefits listed more than just saying that, it's like a complete pharmacy in a bowl.

Maybe Hippocrates was really onto something, hey?

By this time, you may be wondering one of 2 points, if not both.

1. Do I have enough of these ingredients to make my own soup?
2. Why are there still so many pages in this book?

There is still so much to cover.

What you will notice in the ingredients that I have listed is that there are no fillers in them. There's no rice, noodles, tortillas, dumplings, potatoes, turnips…like you may find in the "New and Improved" versions of Chicken Soup, nor even barley, which was said to be in Hippocrates version.

I want to cover fillers for a quick moment and am going to do this with an example. This isn't something that you're not aware of, but just to give an idea why I've excluded the above fillers from the ingredients list that I've used.

Chicken nuggets. Definitely a fan favorite for both adults and children alike and in this, I've grabbed a little nutritional information about these to just compare them to a whole food, equal amount of chicken.

While these ingredients may vary from brand to brand and may be different at each fast-food chain, of the most common I could find, this is what you'd be consuming in a single nugget.

Ingredients: White Boneless Chicken, Water, Vegetable Oil (canola Oil, Corn Oil, Soybean Oil, Hydrogenated Soybean Oil), Enriched Flour (bleached Wheat Flour, Niacin, Reduced Iron, Thiamine Mononitrate, Riboflavin, Folic Acid), Bleached Wheat Flour, Yellow Corn Flour, Vegetable Starch (modified Corn, Wheat, Rice, Pea, Corn), Salt, Leavening (baking Soda, Sodium Aluminum Phosphate, Sodium Acid Pyrophosphate, Calcium Lactate, Monocalcium Phosphate), Spices, Yeast Extract, Lemon Juice Solids, Dextrose, Natural Flavors.

Nutritional Value/Chicken Nugget:
Weight: Approximately 20 grams
Calories: 42.5
Total Fat: 2.5 grams
Total Carbs: 2.5 grams
Protein: 2.25 grams

Compared to equal weight of just the White Boneless Chicken used in them:

Nutritional Value:
Weight: 20 grams
Calories: 22
Total Fat: .25 grams
Total Carbs: ZERO
Protein: 4.62 grams

Summary:

Equal weight of 20 grams of white boneless chicken compared to a chicken nugget, has half of the calories, one tenth of the fat, zero carbohydrates and more than twice the protein, without adding a hydrogenated oil, flour, starch, yeast extract and sugar(dextrose).

While I can be pretty sure that you'd not knowingly add the ingredients of a chicken nugget to richen up your soup, a lot of the benefits that we actually see coming from just working with the basic ingredients is a low-glycemic (how specific foods impact blood sugar levels), meal. I'll get to the specific importance of this later.

From the last few years, we've been misled about the severity of illness and risks from COVID. While the medical professionals would have tried to make you believe that everybody was at risk, this is simply not true. When some of them whittled it down to more specific age groups - 80+ at highest risk, this was only partially true but not for the reason of aging specific.

Our first exposures to COVID were images and video sent from China, people dropping dead in the streets. We heard about the massive amounts of people dying globally, hospitals being overrun with sick people. It was truly mass chaos and a little frightening.

But also, in our first exposure to COVID, there was a list of pre-existing health conditions, chronic in nature, where if you had one of them, you were probably going to have a really tough time with COVID.

High-Risk Conditions:
Hypertension - High Blood Pressure
Cardio-vascular disease
Renal Disease
Diabetes
Respiratory Disease - COPD
Dementia
Stroke
Liver Disease
Immuno-Deficiency Diseases

And what worsened your chances at survival were if you'd had a combination of these, risk increased with each additional. 1 = Bad. 2 = Really Bad. 3+ = Death Sentence!

This has always been the case as in, it's never in the history of modern medicine, not been the case.

The sicker you are, the sicker you are going to get, if you encounter a new virus that your body hadn't already built some immunity to.

In the early days, they couldn't actually even identify the symptoms of COVID, besides giving cold and flu-like symptoms, during cold and flu season. Pure insanity, but what a lot of people don't seem to be understanding is that what we're seeing now in cases of Long-COVID, it's the same. There is no consistency of symptoms, which means that the medical community cannot provide any solutions. I'm going to get to this and it's more than just - Vaccine Injury, and when put together, you might believe it at first, but with some investigation, it'll make more sense.

As the pandemic progressed, the shift in high-risk age seemed to be dropping, the average age of COVID mortality in the early days of COVID was 83. That number declined and now hovers around 79. Addition to this, people with no "Diagnosed" Pre-existing Conditions were dying.

Immunocompromised.
Obesity.
And even some folk who looked to be in rather healthy conditions.

Was COVID getting more lethal?

Diving through the pandemic morbidity and mortality statistics, there didn't seem to be any real pattern, which allowed doctors to promote and people to believe that everybody was at some risk.

And if you really tried to drill into this, it was no easy task, but there had to be something, right?

What do those with chronic illness, the elderly, the obese and those who have been immunocompromised have in common?

That was the question that needed to be answered and this pandemic would have been over as quickly as it began. Strangely enough, this wasn't as tricky as some would have you believe, which is why it's baffling as to why we are still playing this silly game of COVID.

To gain a full understanding of this, you must appreciate that your body works like a hybrid, relying on 2 different forms of energy.
1. Energy that your body uses for function - calories.
2. Energy that your body uses for your immune system - Adenosine Triphosphate (ATP).

And it's this second point that we're going to focus on, for obvious reasons. On a regular basis, our immune system is being employed and doing battle from a number of immune triggers.

Immune Triggers:

Pathogens: The most common trigger for an immune reaction is the presence of pathogens. Pathogens are microorganisms that can cause disease, such as bacteria, viruses, and fungi. When the body detects the presence of these invaders, the immune system launches an immune response to target and eliminate them.

Antigens: Antigens are molecules found on the surface of pathogens or foreign substances that can be recognized by the immune system. Antigens serve as markers that signal the immune system to mount a response. The immune system can recognize antigens as foreign and initiate an immune reaction against them.

Inflammatory Signals: Inflammation is a natural response to injury, infection, or tissue damage. When cells are damaged or infected, they release signaling molecules called cytokines and chemokines. These molecules attract immune cells to the site of infection or injury and trigger an inflammatory response.

Allergens: Allergens are substances that can trigger allergic reactions in individuals with allergies. When the immune system encounters an allergen, it mistakenly identifies it as harmful and launches an immune response, leading to allergy symptoms.

Autoantigens: In some autoimmune diseases, the immune system mistakenly recognizes the body's own tissues and cells as foreign invaders. This results in an immune reaction against self-antigens, leading to tissue damage and autoimmune disease symptoms.

Vaccines: Vaccines contain weakened or inactivated forms of pathogens or parts of pathogens, such as proteins or antigens. When a person receives a vaccine, the immune system is exposed to these antigens and learns to recognize them without causing disease. This prepares the immune system to mount a rapid and effective response if the person is later exposed to the actual pathogen.

Stress and Hormones: Stress and hormones, such as cortisol and adrenaline, can modulate the immune response. Acute stress or the "fight or flight" response can temporarily suppress certain aspects of the immune system, while chronic stress may lead to immune dysfunction.

Injury and Tissue Damage: Physical injury or tissue damage can trigger localized immune responses. The release of damage-associated molecular patterns (DAMPs) from injured cells can activate the immune system and initiate the healing process.

Chemical Irritants: Exposure to certain chemicals, toxins, or irritants can provoke an immune response. For example, inhaling harmful chemicals or toxins can lead to lung inflammation and an immune reaction.

Metabolic Disturbances: Metabolic disorders and imbalances, such as high blood sugar in diabetes, can affect the immune system's function. Chronic metabolic conditions can increase the risk of infections and immune-related complications.

Which, for the most part can all be tucked into 4 main categories - Injury, Poison, Chronic Illness, Bacteria/Virus and the immune response is directly proportional to the severity of the exposure.

If you stub your toe - Immune Reaction.
If you break your toe - More Severe Immune Reaction
If you get run over by a car…you get it.

The point is our immune system is being taxed daily and requires a constant replenishment of energy. The energy that it uses - ATP. When our cells or immune system use that energy, a phosphate molecule is released and available for use, and ATP becomes Adenosine Diphosphate (ADP) - Hydrolysis, and when we need to recharge the ADP back into ATP - Chemiosmotic Phosphorylation.

And the backup charge for converting ADP back into ATP, is phosphocreatine, which is both free-flowing in our bodies, heart and brain - 5%, and the other 95% is stored in our Muscles.

Shortened, energy for function - stored in our fat, energy for our immunity - stored in our muscles, and here's where we get to bring some of this together.
Those with Chronic Illness and who are Immuno-compromised, require a regular and steady supply of phosphocreatine, because they use more of this energy.

Elderly and Obese have a disproportion of body mass to muscle storage, requiring a more regular supply of phosphocreatine - they don't have enough storage for this energy.

Here's the thing, this idea was actually published, as a hypothesis, on April 22, 2020 - on PubMed, under the heading - The powerful immune system against powerful COVID-19 (4 months after the first case of COVID was presumptively detected in North America), assembling information from 19 studies, with the powerful claim, "In this article, we aim to provide a new hypothesis to describe how the repletion of cellular adenosine triphosphate (c-ATP) can promote immunity against COVID-19."

If only there was an abundant source of phosphocreatine available that high risk individuals could benefit from, right?

[Chicken Soup Has Entered the Chat]

In the list of Vitamins, Minerals and Nutrients for each of the Chicken Soup ingredients, Creatine shows up beside Chicken, described in the Amino Acid Benefits: ATP Regeneration: Creatine is best known for its role in the rapid regeneration of adenosine triphosphate (ATP), the primary energy currency of cells.

In addition to this, Chicken also contains the 3 Amino Acids that are the building blocks of Creatine - Arginine, Glycine and Methionine.

This is important for a couple of different reasons, the first and most important is that Creatine has a half-life in the body of about 3 hours. Meaning that after consumption of creatine, whatever your body doesn't use or cannot store, will begin to be excreted. On a daily basis and under regular strain, we use between 1.5 and 2% of our bodies' stored Creatine per day, meaning that we need to replenish this amount and maintain muscle mass in order for this Immune Energy to be available, so when we run out of our consumed or stored sources, we need to be able to fall back on our body being able to create it.

Think about this like you would with your Basal Metabolic Rate, (BMR):

The amount of energy (calories) that an individual's body needs to maintain basic physiological functions while at rest. These functions include breathing, circulation, cell production, and other metabolic activities that are necessary to sustain life. BMR is often expressed as the number of calories burned per day when a person is at complete rest, both physically and mentally.

Factors that Influence BMR:

Body Composition: Lean body mass (muscle) requires more energy to maintain than fat tissue. Therefore, individuals with higher muscle mass tend to have a higher BMR.

Age: BMR typically decreases with age, primarily because muscle mass tends to decrease, and fat mass tends to increase as people get older.

Gender: In general, men tend to have a higher BMR than women, as they often have more muscle mass.

Hormones: Thyroid hormones play a significant role in regulating BMR. An imbalance in thyroid function can lead to changes in BMR.

Genetics: Some individuals may have a naturally higher or lower BMR based on their genetics.

Diet and Nutrition: Extreme calorie restriction or fasting can temporarily lower BMR as the body adapts to conserve energy. Adequate nutrition and regular meals support a healthy BMR.

Health Conditions: Certain medical conditions, such as hyperthyroidism (an overactive thyroid), can increase BMR, while conditions like hypothyroidism (an underactive thyroid) can lower it.

Temperature: Extreme environmental temperatures (very hot or very cold) can affect BMR as the body works to regulate its temperature.

Too few calories consumed per day and we are deficient and need to rely on the stored energy in our bodies - Fat. When we are Calorie Deficient, this can result in a benefit of weight loss.

This is the same sort of process that happens with our immune energy, only when we are Energy Deficient in our immune system, this can result in terrible things happening.

When our bodies are deficient in Creatine by way of consumption, our body's use the creatine stored in our muscles, but this is not an infinite store. To adjust, when our muscles have been fully depleted of this energy required to replenish our immune systems, our body will go into a catabolic state, breaking down into the amino acids they are composed of, in order to create this same energy.

Two of the Amino Acids that can be used to synthesize creatine, are found in our muscles - Arginine and Methionine whereas the collagen in our skin and bones, is made up of about 33% Glycine - the third building block.

Can you see where we are headed here?

Sarcopenia

Muscle Loss: Sarcopenia involves a decrease in the size and number of muscle fibers, resulting in a reduction in muscle mass. This muscle loss is most pronounced in the lower extremities and the muscles responsible for activities like standing, walking, and lifting.

Muscle Strength Reduction: Along with muscle mass loss, there is a decline in muscle strength, which can make it difficult to perform daily tasks, maintain balance, and engage in physical activities.

Reduced Physical Function: Sarcopenia can lead to decreased physical performance and functional limitations, affecting an individual's ability to perform activities of daily living independently.

Increased Risk of Falls: Weakened muscles and decreased strength can lead to an increased risk of falls, which can result in fractures and other injuries, especially in older adults.

Metabolic Changes: Sarcopenia is associated with changes in metabolism, including reduced resting metabolic rate and insulin resistance, which can contribute to weight gain and metabolic disorders.

Contributing Factors:

- **Aging:** Sarcopenia is primarily an age-related condition, with muscle mass and strength naturally declining as individuals get older.
- **Physical Inactivity:** A sedentary lifestyle can accelerate muscle loss and weaken muscles.

- **Poor Nutrition:** Inadequate protein intake, as well as insufficient intake of other nutrients, can contribute to muscle loss.
- **Hormonal Changes:** Changes in hormone levels, such as a decrease in growth hormone and sex hormones, can affect muscle maintenance.
- **Chronic Illness:** Certain chronic conditions, such as cancer, heart disease, and chronic kidney disease, can lead to muscle wasting.
- **Medications:** Some medications can have muscle-wasting side effects.

Cachexia

Unintentional Weight Loss: Cachexia involves substantial, unintentional weight loss, often exceeding 5% of a person's total body weight over a period of six months or less. In some cases, weight loss can be much more dramatic.

Muscle Atrophy: Cachexia is characterized by the loss of both muscle mass (muscle wasting) and fat tissue. Muscle wasting is a prominent feature and contributes to weakness and physical debilitation.

Anorexia: Individuals with cachexia typically experience a loss of appetite (anorexia), which can lead to reduced food intake. This anorexia is often more severe than what is observed in simple malnutrition.

Systemic Inflammation: Chronic diseases associated with cachexia often involve a state of chronic inflammation. The body's immune response and production of inflammatory molecules can contribute to muscle breakdown and metabolic changes.

Fatigue and Weakness: Cachexia can result in extreme fatigue, weakness, and a decline in physical function, which further impairs an individual's quality of life.

Contributing factors:

- Increased production of inflammatory cytokines, such as tumor necrosis factor-alpha (TNF-alpha) and interleukin-6 (IL-6).
- Altered metabolism, including increased resting energy expenditure.

- Abnormalities in muscle protein turnover and muscle protein synthesis.
- Changes in hormone levels, including elevated levels of cortisol.
- Loss of appetite-regulating hormones, such as ghrelin.

Summary:

As we get older, our skin gets more wrinkled, our hair grays and falls out and our bones get weaker and with limited movement, muscle mass is depleted, organs less efficient, if not damaged by a life of exposure. Throw in chronic illness, injury, exposure to toxins and things aren't looking good.

Add all of that in, and while we were subjected to colder climates, closed air spaces with exposure to viruses and bacteria (typical respiratory virus season), and we've got a perfect storm.

Again, this didn't change with COVID, this has always been the case.

Let's recap up to this point.

Things that negatively impact our immune systems:

- Allergens.
- Autoantigens.
- Vaccines.
- Stress and Hormones.
- Injury and Tissue Damage.
- Chemical Irritants.
- Metabolic Disturbances:
- Physical Inactivity.

- Poor Nutrition.
- Hormonal Changes.
- Chronic Illness.
- Medications.

And if you look on this list to the words in bold, one thing that you may realize is that these were all included in recommendations, protocols, and mandates to keep us safe.

Vaccines - stressing the body and forcing an immune reaction; Stress - fear spread throughout media 24/7 for 3 years; Injury and tissue Damage - side effects from the vaccines causing Myocarditis; Chemical Irritants - washing hands with alcohol every 5 feet in public; Metabolic Disturbances and Physical Inactivity - lockdown measures restricting movement and closing down gyms playgrounds and parks; Poor Nutrition - keeping fast food restaurants and liquor stores open; Medications - prescribing an additional - at home therapy, Paxlovid, which ended up resulting in Rebound Cases of COVID.

Things that we can do to assist and improve our immune systems:

- Eat Chicken Soup.

And if you look at this one item, it provides a vast array of immune supporting vitamins, minerals, nutrients and amino acids, works to replenish electrolytes while keeping us hydrated, recharges immune batteries, helps maintain muscle mass, lowers inflammation and as an added benefit, tastes pretty good.

Makes a pretty good case for stick'n with chick'n, doesn't it?

Thermogenesis

How does chicken soup help keep you warm?

Sure, having a hot tea or cup of cocoa, will raise the body temperature in the same way as having a belly full of hot soup, but there really is a little more that the ingredients in chicken soup offer. Like sweating in the summer to help keep cool, our bodies have evolved to warm up during the cooler climates. This process is called Thermogenesis - a physiological process where we generate heat.

Types of Thermogenesis:

Basal Metabolic Rate (BMR) Thermogenesis: This is the heat produced by the body at rest to maintain basic physiological functions, such as breathing, circulation, and cell metabolism. BMR accounts for the majority of daily energy expenditure and is influenced by factors like age, gender, muscle mass, and genetics.

Diet-Induced Thermogenesis (DIT): Also known as the thermic effect of food (TEF), DIT is the increase in metabolic rate that occurs after eating due to the digestion, absorption, and metabolism of food. Different macronutrients have varying thermogenic effects, with protein having a higher thermic effect compared to carbohydrates and fats.

Exercise-Induced Thermogenesis (EIT): When you engage in physical activity, your body generates heat as a byproduct of muscle contraction. The intensity and duration of exercise influence the extent of EIT. High-intensity exercise, such as weightlifting and sprinting, can produce more heat than low-intensity activities.

Non-Shivering Thermogenesis (NST): NST is a specialized form of thermogenesis primarily associated with brown adipose tissue (brown fat). Brown fat is rich in mitochondria and is capable of generating heat without muscle movement.

Adaptive Thermogenesis: This type of thermogenesis occurs in response to environmental conditions. When exposed to cold temperatures, for example, the body may increase thermogenesis to maintain core temperature. Shivering is a common form of adaptive thermogenesis.

While most of these are what our bodies can do naturally, the ingredients in Chicken Soup lend themselves to 2 of these types:
1. Diet-Induced.
2. Non-Shivering.

Diet-Induced Thermogenesis:

Yes, the consumption of all foods has a thermogenic effect. Food Energy is Measured in Calories, the amount of energy required to raise the temperature of 1 gram of water by 1 degree celsius. If you eat more calories, you get warmer, is something we all know. That's why eating a large pizza sitting in the sun is a terrible idea, whereas the benefit of this many calories on a cold day, may serve to keep you warm.

However, in the previously listed example of increasing calorie count in a chicken nugget by way of fillers and other ingredients, while there may be a greater thermogenic response by your body (making you feel warmer), these fillers don't just increase your body temperature, they may also cause or increase the inflammation inside of your body, triggering a greater immune response.

Inflammatory foods, as in food items that can increase the amount of inflammation inside of your body are what we see as typical type fillers in processed food items but also in traditional meals and recipes as well. These items are cost effective, make for easy storage and to a certain extent, can add some flavor, texture and heartiness to your meals.

An example of inflammatory foods are any flour based item, like breads, cereals and cake - specific to a bowl of soup may look like dumplings or noodles. Typically made from refined white flour, may also contain sugar, seed and hydrogenated or seed oils.

What these do is create a spike in blood sugar which releases proinflammatory molecules called cytokines, a part of the body's immune response and

are involved in inflammation. Symptoms of respiratory viruses, such as a runny or stuffy nose, sore throat, and cough, are the result of the body's immune response to a viral infection and Cytokines play a significant role in this immune response and can contribute to the
severity of the reaction moving from Asymptomatic to full-blown Man Cold! Increased blood sugar can increase cytokines, which will increase the reaction inside of your body. While the initial reaction may be due to your body naturally fighting a virus, they are worsened by creating an environment where this inflammation is being fed through the consumption of inflammatory foods in much the same way fires get larger when you add gasoline.

Addition to this, high sugar intake can contribute to formation of advanced glycation end products - (AGEs). These are compounds formed when sugars react with proteins or fats in the body, can accumulate and promote oxidative stress inside the body.

Lastly, additional calories added by way of inflammatory food promote obesity, which in turn increases body mass while not lending itself to the size of storage - muscles - for energy for our immune systems.

Okay. You're probably not going to get fat from a bowl of soup but at the same time, limiting your calorie intake will reduce your blood sugar response, which in turn will reduce cytokine/immune response which will reduce the severity of symptoms during illness.

To put this in a way that's more easily understood, our bodies adjust to both burning calories (Basal Metabolic Rate), in the same way that it adjusts to our immune reaction. For the most part, barring chronic conditions, these are kept in check through our ability to adapt to minor changes while being in a state of homeostasis - self-regulating processes. When these are tested, they can result in minor reactions but typically we are able to maintain pain and symptom free lives.

When we introduce major shifts in our day to day lives, they can have profound impacts on our body.

It's like this.

While you are living your everyday life, you maintain some quality of foods, probably some exercise and a regular sleep pattern. This is the foundation of your immune system - regular and consistent: Diet + Exercise + Sleep = Healthy Immune System.

When you decide that it's time for a vacation, all of these are in perfect check. Maybe not the most ideal, but to your existence they are homeostatic - your immune system comfort zone. At this point, your immune system is capable of handling the viruses that you are exposed to on your flight, asymptomatic.

While you are on vacation, you have disrupted everything that keeps your immunity in check under the basic premise of maximizing your holiday. You eat foods that are foreign to you, you slack off on a regular exercise routine, you are not sleeping in your own bed and you are not maintaining the same healthy sleep patterns you have at home. You've been stressing your body since you woke up and packed your suitcase, you've dealt with stress parking at the airport, finding your gate, checking your bag…there really is a massive amount of stress that we put our bodies through to "Take a break".

Your immune system has suffered through a week of hell for you to have some tan lines, a few selfies and bragging rights.

On the flight home, you are exposed to another batch of bacteria, germs and viruses and with your now weakened immune system, increased blood sugars, depleted immune energy, the cytokine response is now greater, meaning that you feel like trash or are completely laid out for a week in recovery - full on symptomatic.

Add in chronic inflammatory conditions, which may already be taxing your immune energy and things are a lot worse.

But what does this all have to do with being warmed by a bowl of chicken soup, you might be asking?

Good question if you did.

There are properties inside of the ingredients of Chicken Soup which will lend itself to thermogenesis - being warmed, without adding in higher glycemic or inflammatory foods that can create more profound immune/cytokine responses.

Piperine:

A component of Black Pepper, mentioned earlier, can create a thermogenic effect through several mechanisms:

Increased Metabolism: Piperine is believed to stimulate the metabolism by increasing the production of certain enzymes involved in digestion and metabolism. One such enzyme is called thermogenic co-factor 1 (Thermofin), which is involved in the breakdown of fat cells.

Enhanced Nutrient Absorption: Piperine has been shown to enhance the absorption of various nutrients, including vitamins and minerals, from the gastrointestinal tract. This enhanced nutrient absorption can indirectly contribute to a thermogenic effect by improving the body's overall metabolic processes.

Activation of Brown Adipose Tissue (Brown Fat): Brown adipose tissue, or brown fat, is a type of fat tissue that can generate heat when activated. It plays a role in thermogenesis. Some research suggests that piperine may activate brown fat, leading to an increase in energy expenditure and heat production.

Improved Insulin Sensitivity: Piperine may help improve insulin sensitivity, allowing the body to use glucose more efficiently for energy. Enhanced insulin sensitivity can contribute to better metabolic function and thermogenesis.

Fat Mobilization: Piperine has been shown to influence the expression of genes involved in lipid metabolism. This may lead to increased fat mobilization and utilization for energy, potentially contributing to a thermogenic effect.

Neurotransmitter Regulation: Piperine may influence neurotransmitters in the brain, such as dopamine and serotonin, which can impact mood and appetite regulation. These neurotransmitters can play a role in energy balance and thermogenesis.

Piperine only makes up between 5-9% of Black Pepper, so while you may not realize the full effects and benefits of piperine, it is undeniable that adding a little more pepper to your soup, will cause you to sweat a little more.

Non-Shivering Thermogenesis:

Have you ever heard that babies can't shiver?

If you haven't up until now, you have now. You can check it out, it's true.

Yes, they do get cold and yes, they will also get goosebumps, but they don't actually shiver. The primary reason for this is because the mechanisms responsible for shivering are not as well-developed in infants, but some additional reasons for this may be:

Muscle Mass: Shivering involves the rapid contraction and relaxation of skeletal muscles to generate heat. Newborns and young infants have significantly less muscle mass compared to adults. Their muscle development is still in progress, and their muscles are not as well-coordinated, making it challenging for them to shiver effectively.

Limited Fat Stores: Shivering is often preceded by the depletion of glycogen (stored carbohydrate) in the muscles. In adults, the breakdown of glycogen can fuel shivering. Infants, however, have limited glycogen stores. Instead, **they rely more on brown adipose tissue (brown fat) for non-shivering thermogenesis,** as mentioned in the previous response. Brown fat is more active in generating heat in response to cold in infants.

Thermoregulation: Newborns and young infants have a more challenging time regulating their body temperature compared to adults. They can lose heat rapidly through their relatively large surface area compared to their body mass. To compensate for this, they use mechanisms like non-shivering thermogenesis through brown adipose tissue and adjusting blood flow to conserve heat.

Neurological Development: The control and coordination of muscle activity, including shivering, are complex processes that rely on the maturity of the nervous system. In newborns and infants, the nervous system is still developing, which affects their ability to initiate and sustain coordinated muscle contractions for shivering.

Temperature Sensitivity: While infants can sense changes in temperature, their ability to sense and respond to temperature changes may not be as finely tuned as in adults. Their body temperature regulatory mechanisms are still maturing.

While most of these are theoretical, only one of these really sticks out as being most plausible, to me - Brown Fat Activation - much the same as was mentioned in the effects of piperine.

Shivering is an involuntary and rather violent process and becomes even more so with illness or a virus. Take the sniffles, a fever, sore throat and then go into a wave of shivering and you can appreciate why you have no actual appreciation for this body warming mechanism.

Simply put, it sucks!

In infants, can you imagine the shock and damage that could be done by full on shivering to these developing banks of cellular information whose only early purposes are eating, pooping, crying and surviving?

Think - Shaken Baby Syndrome!

Maybe it wouldn't be this traumatic or terrifying but at the same time, what we have to understand is that it is possible for our body to create thermogenic heat, without the violent reaction - Non-Shivering Thermogenesis through Brown Fat Activation.

How does this work?

Like this:

Brown Fat Activation: When brown fat is activated, either in response to cold temperatures or other stimuli, it generates heat through a process called thermogenesis. This heat production is achieved by the activation of a protein called Uncoupling Protein 1 (UCP1) present in brown fat cells.

Burning Calories: The primary function of brown fat is to burn calories to produce heat. Instead of storing energy like white fat, which stores excess calories in the form of triglycerides, brown fat expends energy by converting it into heat. This means that when brown fat is active, it consumes calories.

White Fat Utilization: Brown fat can also have an indirect effect on white fat. When brown fat burns calories for heat, it can draw on stored triglycerides from white fat tissue for a source of energy.

Thermogenesis Summarized

Brown fat burns white fat to create thermogenesis.

As infants, we have larger stores of Brown Fat and as we get older, we lose or deplete these same stores - replacing them more with Stored Energy - White Fat, (love handles and beer bellies). A large part of this is due to modernization and adaptation to modern conveniences of warmer thermal clothing and climate-controlled environments.

We have heaters in our homes, our cars, our workplaces.

We have warmer coats, socks, boots and gloves.

Our body no longer has the same necessity for maintaining brown fat, so it whittles down and we have less ability to burn white fat. Want to know the reasons why obesity is becoming more rampant?

This is definitely a part of it!

Cold Adaptation can help generate more brown fat and make us more able to adjust to colder temperatures through this non-shivering, non-violent process of thermogenesis, but taking a cold shower when you are already shivering is actually a terrible idea - will stress your body and could create an even stronger cytokine/immune reaction.

The process is Cold Adaptation, as in after a single cold shower you will not generate enough brown fat to be of any great benefit, this comes from regular exposure to colder temperatures.

Think of this like bodybuilding.

One day at the gym will not have that profound of an impact on sculpting your body; a regular pattern of working out, will.

And how does this have anything to do with Chicken Soup?

Another excellent question!

In the Amino Acids listed for Chicken, I'd broken out the Branched Chain Amino Acids (BCAAs) and their specific benefit on building muscle and I'd also listed Hydroxymethylbutyrate - HMB, a chemical that is made when the body breaks down Leucine - one of the Branched Chain Amino Acids.

In addition to performing a number of additional benefits previously stated, HMB influences fat metabolism and increases fat oxidation - which are some of the processes involved in Non-Shivering Thermogenesis.

Essentially, HMB will in some of the same ways act like Brown Adipose Tissue in creating the same effects of Non-Shivering Thermogenesis that you'd get from Cold Adaptation. You will still feel the cold, but your body will be more efficient at creating a thermogenic effect, without the requirement of violent shivering.

Summarized:

2 components of the ingredients of Chicken Soup - Piperine and HMB, work to activate your brown adipose tissue as well as increase fat oxidation to create a thermogenic warming effect - helping to soothe you and reduce suffering from the violent reaction of shivering. These are also 2 components that do not greatly increase your blood sugar levels and won't have the same negative impacts on your cytokine/immune response in the way that processed foods and sugars will.

Are you going to get all of these benefits out of a pot of Chicken Soup?

Honestly, it's unlikely.

But there is still more to cover on Chicken Soup, moving into, is it a soup or is it a broth?

Is it a Soup or is it a Broth?

It's both.

Chicken Soup can be served as both a soup, hearty and full of vegetables as a meal in a bowl but when you are sick is typically served as a broth, suited for sipping out of a cup and there are very distinct differences to what it will lend under both conditions.

Firstly, as a bowl of soup:

The heartier the soup, the greater the nutritional impact on your body - of course keeping the fillers and inflammatory foods low. It's a great way to replenish and maintain the majority of vitamins and nutrients in your body, the skin from the chicken lending a fat source for your fat-soluble vitamins - A, D, E and K, the Amino Acid profile of chicken works to improve your muscle mass, reduce muscle catabolism and provide the energy for your immune system - creatine.

As a broth:

Inside of a broth, you will see very trace amounts of vitamins and nutrients, smaller on the amino acid side of things, perhaps little to no creatine and may only get a little flavoring from the herbs and vegetables in the ingredients. On the surface, it may seem as though there may not be any benefits from this with maybe the exception of hydration, however, there is a lot of complexity to just this.

In progressing from scarcity to abundance, we have come to accept that more is always better, especially when it comes to providing benefits and, on the nutritional/consumption side of benefits, we've come to accept generic values called Recommended Daily Allowances (RDA) for dietary recommendations.

This has been hijacked and is used to exploit base knowledge and for commercial purposes. While these values have been broken down by age stratification, height and weight references and even down to sex, the amount of information inside of RDAs would be almost impossible to adhere to as a set lifestyle decision as well as too time consuming to monitor. Addition to this, RDAs assume that while you may not be in perfect health, you are in average health - free from chronic illness or inflammatory disease.

Look at just the advertising around Vegetable Cocktails - claiming to contain 2 full servings of vegetables in an 8-ounce glass.

How many brands of orange juice are now fortified with Vitamin D?

Have you seen the size of the vitamin and supplement section inside of pharmacies and grocery stores?

Health has become a multibillion-dollar industry of its own, but how much of this has been hijacked and bastardized to sell you more product?

How much of this is actually of benefit?

Let's explore.

When you go to the pharmacy or pharmacy aisles in your grocer and you are looking for pain relief, you can find both regular and extra strength. Using Ibuprofen as an example, when you buy regular strength, you get a 200mg pill and when you get the extra strength version, you get a 400mg pill.

It's not that one works faster or harder, it's all to do with the size of the pill.

If you don't suffer from chronic or regular pain, you may opt for the smaller size and double the dosage in your self-medicating plan for pain management. If you do suffer from a chronic inflammatory condition or are in extreme pain, you'll buy the extra strength to not have to take as many pills.

Vitamins and supplements are the same, only without the additional descriptors of Regular or Extra Strength. As an example, you can find Vitamin C from

300 mg to 1000 mg as well as it being folded into a smaller quantity in a multivitamin, but never see the words - Regular or Extra Strength - Vitamin C.

How much do you need per day?

This too is complicated because under certain extenuating circumstances, your body may require larger doses. Leafing back to the Benefits of Vitamin C, you will all of these benefits:

Antioxidant Activity, Immune System Support, Collagen Production, Skin Health, Wound Healing, Iron Absorption, Eye Health, Stress Reduction, Heart Health, Antiviral and Antimicrobial Effects, Cancer Prevention, Brain Health.

These are all pretty important things, so we should probably be taking a lot of Vitamin C, right?

According to the Mayo Clinic, the RDA for Vitamin C is 75 mg per day for women and 90 mg per day for men. Have you ever seen Vitamin C come in either of 75 or 90 mg sizes?

The smallest size you'll most likely find is 4-8 x greater. Given its importance in the body and low toxicity, you can take as much as you want with little to no side effects. Vitamin/supplement proponents will recommend that you actually take this to 'bowel tolerance' - a side effect you hit at 6000 - 8000 mg in a sitting, where you are afraid to walk past the bathroom and may spend a good portion of your day with a sick stomach and leaky stool.

Why the hell would you do this?

I don't have a good answer for you.

Let's look at another example - Vitamin D.

Vitamin D comes in as small of size as 1,000 International Units (IU) and goes up to 10,000.

Benefits of Vitamin D:

Bone Health, Immune system Support, Mood Regulation, Heart Health, Cancer Prevention, Support for Immune Function, Weight Management, Brain Health, Skin Health and Regulation of Calcium and Phosphorus.

Again, sounds pretty important and dosing may be specific to your particular condition.

If you're old and want less wrinkles and a better immune system - take more, right?

Mayo Clinic puts the RDA for Vitamin D at 400 IU for children up to the age of 12 months, 60 IU for ages 1-70 and 800 IU for 80+, as in, the smallest size you can most likely find of Vitamin D, is more than you need to take if you are over the age of 80.

Is the Mayo Clinic completely out to lunch on these RDAs?

Why have a 10,000 IU sized version of something that you may only require in 1/10th of this dosing size?

Throughout COVID, we'd seen that being deficient in Vitamin D put you into a higher risk category for the most severe outcome of COVID, being death. For months, every social media platform was inundated with studies and proponents of Vitamin D screaming from the rooftops to take Vitamin D and a lot of these, in greater quantities that even supersede the 10K IU.

I am not going to try and make the argument that Vitamin D is not important. I am not even going to go into the "Correlation doesn't mean Causation", conversation. Under a lot of healthcare systems, the cost for testing for a Vitamin D deficiency so far exceeds the cost of supplementation of Vitamin D, that if you have symptoms that mimic Vitamin D deficiency, it's recommended that you spend the $10, get a bottle of the supplemental version and start taking them.

How much and for how long, is what I question.

Before Vitamin Supplements were available, we had to rely on being out in the sun to get our RDA and in the cooler months with shorter days, what we could get from food. Vitamin D being a fat-soluble vitamin is only available in fatty fish/animal-based proteins and cannot be supplemented through vegetables.

Let's drill this out.

A Large Chicken egg, depending on your method of cooking, has between 40 and 50 IU of Vitamin D. If you are between the age of 1-70, you need 800 IUs of Vitamin D according to the Mayo Clinic - meaning that if eggs were your only option, you'd need to consume between 16 and 20 eggs per day. Proponents of Vitamin D and the largest sized pill available are at 10K IUs per day, meaning that if eggs were your only option, you'd need to consume between 200 and 250, PER DAY.

Never in the history of the planet would you have ever conceived that a person living in the prairies or away from open waters and away from fish (richest sources of Vitamin D), would need to consume 17 Dozen Eggs PER DAY to be healthy during the winter months. It can't be done!

Another rich source of Vitamin D - a 219g porkchop/blade with the bone contains 87.6 IUs. Could you eat 10 of these?

How about 114 of them?

Per Day?

So why the hell would somebody recommend this much Vitamin D?

Again, I don't have a good answer for you.

Important to note, while there is Vitamin D in Chicken nor any of the other ingredients in Chicken Soup, the trace amounts are too small to be of any value and the reason that I never included it in the Vitamins nor Benefits section.

All of this just to explain that as far as we've come on nutritional information and as widely as it's been made available, there is still a lot more to uncover and unconfuse, especially seeing that a bowl of Chicken Soup - Broth, while it may contain a vast array of essential vitamins, minerals, nutrients and amino acids they too are in trace quantities that may seem too small to benefit from.

You may be a little disappointed in where this has all come to.

This is a lot of reading to realize that there may in fact be No Benefits to Eating Chicken Soup and that Hippocrates may have been a 5th Century BC, Quack.

You may at this point even feel like you've been duped.

Don't.

I'm not finished yet.

Less is More

You may have heard these words thrown around, "less is more". When you do, you may be of the mindset that you are about to be had, and even up to this point in the book, you've read or scanned over around 20,000 words, you may be of the mindset that more isn't necessarily more either.

Here's the thing, when we go back to the things that trigger our immune system, depleting immune energy that could be used to fight off 'the sniffles', what we need to understand is that if we have **less** immune triggers, we have **more** immune energy.

Again, Immune Triggers being:

Pathogens, Antigens, **Inflammatory Signals**, Allergens, Autoantigens, **Vaccines**, **Stress and Hormones**, Injury and Tissue Damage, Chemical Irritants, Metabolic Disturbances.

But also include the contributing factors of the catabolic processes of Sarcopenia and Cachexia:

Aging, Physical Inactivity, Poor Nutrition, Chronic Illness, **Medications, Increased production of inflammatory cytokines, altered metabolism**, Abnormalities in muscle protein turnover and muscle protein synthesis, **Changes in hormone levels, including elevated levels of cortisol**, Loss of appetite-regulating hormones, such as ghrelin.

Not all of these are inside of your control. You are not making the conscious decision to get cancer or slip on the ice and break your leg. You're not necessarily in control of your aging process, pathogens nor allergens.

But instead of looking at all of the things that you cannot control, it's important to look at what you can - mitigation of damage, by way of creating conditions that will not work to deplete your energy nor damage your body further.

A reasonable example of this, if you want to protect your liver from Cirrhosis (scar tissue replacing healthy liver tissue), don't drink alcoholic beverages.

If you want to protect your liver from Non-Alcoholic Fatty Liver Disease (NALFD), cut out the carbs, sugars, and processed foods.

I know, this is easier said than done.

However, mitigation doesn't require perfection, at least this is what I tell myself and, as it turns out, it's actually true.

Can you have a cheat day on a diet and still lose weight?
Yes.

Can you still have the odd day of imbibing and still maintain healthy liver function?
Also, yes.

Our bodies adapt and they are able to heal to certain extents.

If you cut yourself, the wound will heal. Break a bone, it will heal. Burn yourself, it will heal...

All of these and a lot more are natural processes and while we may not heal to perfection, we can heal to levels of comfort or at least minimize discomfort and maintain function. Where we get bogged down with this is through the introduction of what we have now come to understand as modernized Healthcare being Pharmacare.

Like the ideas behind pain mitigation through ibuprofen in taking a larger dosage dependent on pain levels, or supplementation by way of over consuming realistic amounts of essential vitamins and nutrients, we do similar through what we've come to understand as Medicine.

Take More for More Benefits.

And from my examples on both Vitamin C and Vitamin D, what you may have gathered is that there could be some negative implications from this to unreasonable quantities to try and achieve benefits. With supplementation, there is very little risk.

LD50 of Vitamin C is 11,900 mgs per kilogram.

LD50 is a measure used during experimentation to establish how much exposure to a certain chemical will kill 50% of the test subjects (rats). On average, the LD50 of Vitamin C would mean that a rat would have to consume 3.5% of its body weight in Vitamin C before it becomes lethal.

Extending this out, if you weighed 150 lbs., you would need to consume 5.25 lbs. of Ascorbic Acid - Vitamin C before you'd hit lethal dosage. The average meal is 1.2 pounds, 3.6 total pounds for your daily consumption based on 3 meals per day and considering that you'd begin to lose bowel control after consuming 8,000 mgs of Vitamin C, consumption of 5.25 lbs. is impossible.

Please do not try and prove me wrong.

The difference comes into play when we are adding chemicals that are foreign to our bodies (toxins), potential for side-effects or adverse reactions and their Lethal Dosage - pharmaceuticals. Add to this, how pharmaceuticals may react with other pharmaceuticals for lethality.

Adverse Drug Reactions, according to the most recent studies that I could find, suggest that between 5 and 10% of patients may be hospitalized due to drug interactions/overdoses and that this may be as high as the 4th leading cause of death, in westernized countries. The important thing to note here is that medicine today isn't actually a cure for anything. Masking symptoms and lessening severity of disease or discomfort are their only benefit but come with a wide range of reactions that can worsen health and lead to muscle and bone loss, as stated in the contributing factors of sarcopenia and cachexia.

You've been there. Watching TV, maybe listening to the radio and a pharmaceutical commercial comes on.
"Ask your doctor if [insert random pharmaceutical] is right for you."

"For what?" You may ask…

Do you suffer from an upset stomach, abdominal pain, constipation, diarrhea, fatigue, feeling confused or dizzy, feeling thirsty and dry mouth, headaches, increased urination, lightheadedness, muscle cramps or weak muscles.

It's good news for you, my friend!

[Insert random pharmaceutical], is the answer to all of your problems, the only issue is, that there may be some side effects and those side effects may include but are not limited to: upset stomach, abdominal pain, constipation, diarrhea, fatigue, feeling confused or dizzy, feeling thirsty and dry mouth, headaches, increased urination, lightheadedness, muscle cramps or weak muscles.

Dear Lord! How did we achieve the status of being highest on the food chain with this sort of logic?

In the list of chronic conditions that lead to the highest risk for mortality with respiratory viruses, there are hundreds of pharmaceuticals that you may be taking. When you have more than a single chronic condition, there are hundreds of combinations of medications that you may be prescribed. The potential for risk is greatly increased with each additional drug you take as is the damage that can be done to your body. Throw in a respiratory virus, add in a vaccine, take a pain med for your headache and we're lucky to see death by prescription/overdose has only made it to #4 on the list of leading causes of mortality.

Making matters worse is the fact that the LD50 of most drugs is considerably lower than that of Vitamin C, or any other of the listed vitamins and minerals in Chicken Soup - which has only barely touched on the Adverse Reactions to these, not only being death.

The most common adverse reactions to prescription pharmaceuticals are:

Gastrointestinal Symptoms: These may include nausea, vomiting, diarrhea, constipation, and stomach pain. Many medications can irritate the gastrointestinal tract.

Drowsiness or Fatigue: Some drugs, particularly those that affect the central nervous system, can cause drowsiness, sedation, or fatigue.

Allergic Reactions: Allergic reactions to medications can range from mild skin rashes and itching to more severe symptoms like hives, swelling, and difficulty breathing. Anaphylaxis is a rare but life-threatening allergic reaction.

Dizziness or Lightheadedness: Some drugs can cause dizziness or a feeling of being lightheaded, which can increase the risk of falls and accidents.

Headache: Headaches are a common side effect of many medications.

Dry Mouth: Some drugs can lead to decreased saliva production, resulting in a dry mouth.

Weight Gain or Weight Loss: Certain medications can lead to changes in appetite and weight.

Skin Reactions: Skin reactions may include rashes, itching, redness, or photosensitivity (increased sensitivity to sunlight).

Changes in Blood Pressure: Some medications can cause either an increase or a decrease in blood pressure.

Changes in Blood Sugar: Certain drugs, such as those used to treat diabetes or corticosteroids, can affect blood sugar levels.

Changes in Kidney or Liver Function: Some medications may affect the function of these organs, which may be monitored through blood tests.

Muscle Pain or Weakness: Statins, a class of drugs used to lower cholesterol, are known to sometimes cause muscle pain or weakness.

Cognitive Effects: Some medications can impact cognitive function, leading to memory problems, confusion, or difficulty concentrating.

Mood Changes: Certain drugs can affect mood and may lead to symptoms like anxiety, depression, or mood swings.

Sexual Dysfunction: Some medications can cause sexual side effects, including decreased libido, erectile dysfunction, or changes in menstrual cycles.

Whereas for the vaccinations that were introduced for COVID, there were a solid 8 pages of tiny writing with no description and millions of these adverse reactions reported in just North America alone and again, these ranged from soreness or swelling at the injection site through to death as well. In this, what is important to realize is that the vaccines alone were most likely NOT the direct cause of mortality, in the same way the COVID was never the direct cause of fatality.

The majority of the adverse reactions listed from prescriptions or vaccinations, is a physical injury which triggers an immune response. The severity of this response is directly dependent on current health and pre-existing conditions, in the same way as the consumption of inflammatory foods can lead to a more extreme cytokine/immune reaction.

Simply put.

If you are already ill with one or more of the pre-existing health conditions that put you in the high risk for severity of COVID, (as would to any additional taxation on your immune system), and were taking a medication that was further depleting your immune energy, came into contact with a virus - you are going to have a really bad time with this.

And I cannot overstate the importance of what all of this means.

When we look now and see the amount of "Long COVID" cases and why doctors cannot figure out how to deal with this because of the inconsistency of the symptoms, what you have to realize is that by lowering your immune system with a vaccine that has 8 pages of adverse reactions and are already taking medication that has a laundry list of its own and you come into contact with any respiratory virus or bacteria, how will you know which of these is causing the Longer Symptoms?

Throughout several conversations with vaccinated and unvaccinated people who are claiming that they have Long COVID, what I've gleaned from these conversations is that their symptoms aren't actually symptoms of COVID, but in a quick dive into the analytics of this, they are seemingly the side effects listed with their existing prescriptions.

Let's take a look.

Correlative Analysis

If you have a look at the most common symptoms of Long COVID, you'll see the following:

Breathing Difficulties
Cognitive Issues
Fatigue
GI Issues
Hair Loss
Headaches
Loss of Taste or Smell
Mood Changes
Muscle and Joint Pain
Skin Rashes
Sleep Disturbances
Temperature Dysregulation

Some of these are easy to accept as symptoms or carry over symptoms of a respiratory virus but others, not so much. 7 out of 12 of these don't seem cross over with COVID are:

Cognitive Issues
Hair Loss
Mood Changes
Muscle and Joint Pain
Skin Rashes
Sleep Disturbances
Temperature Dysregulation

From here, if you were to analyze the prescriptions that may cause these as side effects, the type of prescriptions that seemingly overlaps these leftover symptoms of Long COVID are antidepressants.

And if you drill into this further, what you'd find for a more complete list of side effects from antidepressants are:
Breathing Difficulties
Cognitive Issues
Fatigue
GI Issues
Hair Loss
Headaches
Loss of Taste or Smell
Mood Changes
Muscle and Joint Pain
Skin Rashes
Sleep Disturbances
Temperature Dysregulation

While correlation doesn't necessarily mean causation, you'd have to at very least be a little curious as to why all of the most common symptoms of Long COVID are the same as the side effects from Antidepressants.

What makes this most troubling is the rate of increase in Antidepressant from 2020 through to 2023, globally. While it's hard to pinpoint an average some interesting statistics that I've come across are:

- 1:4 college students are taking antidepressants. (US - 2023)
- An increase in antidepressants in people under 19 years old from 15.9% in 2018 to 19.3% in 2022. (Canada)
- An increase in Antidepressants in seniors went from 22.3% in 2019 to 23.4% in 2021. (Canada)
- Antidepressant prescribing increases by 35% in six years - prescriptions of antidepressants rose by 5.1% in 2021/2022, the sixth consecutive annual increase. (United States)

This is a little scary, isn't it?

Now, if you took this same list of symptoms from Long COVID, being the exact same as potential side effects from Antidepressants and compared this to the 8 pages of side effects from COVID vaccinations, what do you think you'd find?

Amazingly coincidental, these same symptoms show up in various forms.

You may be wondering why the side effects from Antidepressants only appear after COVID or after having been vaccinated for COVID or a combination of them both, if there is in fact any correlation. While I won't try and definitively state a correlation, one possible explanation is that in an otherwise healthy individual who has been taking these prescribed treatments that have known side effects, is already taking a hit to their immune system, and slowly depleting their immune energy. When you add in additional immune triggers be them from COVID itself or having been vaccinated, additional triggers present, and the condition worsens to a more noticeable degree. If the amount of immune energy that's been added back is still less than the amount required, there is a persistent problem that now exists in a more severe form. Chronically taking the same medication that causes persistent symptoms now creates a chronic problem.

You cannot medicate yourself out of a condition that medication may have been responsible for getting you into.

This doesn't touch on the possible reasons for more people dying following weaker variants of COVID after multiple vaccinations and bouts with COVID, but maybe there is more to this story too.

This doesn't touch on the possible reasons for more people dying following weaker variants of COVID after multiple vaccinations and bouts with COVID, but maybe there is more to this story too.

Remember the conditions that put you at high risk from COVID?

Remember how many different types of prescriptions you can get for these?

Imagine having 3(+) pre-existing conditions, taking an antidepressant, because at this point, why wouldn't you be, taking 3 medications for the 3 conditions you have, getting vaccinated and then still getting COVID.

While it's hard to imaging 3 pre-existing conditions, for 3 pre-existing conditions, a report that was published by the Canadian Institute for Health Information in October of 2022 showed that 24.6% of Females and 23.3% of Males - aged 65 and older, were prescribed with 10 or more drug classes, in 2021.

10 or more prescription medications.

For those over the age of 85, the number increased to 36.4%, as in, 1 in 3 Canadians over the age of 85 are taking 10 or more prescriptions. Can you even imagine the overlap of adverse reactions to these, before you added in a vaccination with 8 pages of its own adverse reaction, during flu season?

It gets worse. In the same study it showed that 66% of seniors in Long Term Care were on Antidepressants, 40% on Antipsychotics and about 22% on Benzodiazepines. Added together, that's 128%, meaning that there are people in LTC that are on a mixture of 2 or more of these, inside of the 10(+) prescriptions they are taking.

Whatever adverse reactions they could be having, are completely covered up because these unfortunate souls are little more than walking zombies.

Special Note - Adverse Reactions to Chicken Soup, do not exist.

Back to When Less Becomes More

But when does less become more?

You are sharp, my friend and I'm glad that you asked and that you're here to keep this conversation flowing. Just imagine me prattling on about anything other than Chicken Soup in a book devoted to Chicken Soup that doesn't even have a recipe for Chicken Soup.

Like leaving out inflammatory foods from your Chicken Soup or leaving out most of the solid contents from your Chicken Soup and only consuming the broth, what you are doing is not triggering a spike in blood sugars additional cytokine/immune responses.

When you are sick, you're not much in the mood for eating a weighty meal and maybe not much in the mood for eating at all, and this is okay. For how long?

As long as it can take, really.

In diet and nutrition, one of the myths that we've come to believe is that we need those 3 meals per day consuming 3.6 pounds of food. We don't. While we do have a base requirement for energy to maintain basic physiological functions our body has already got this stored by way of fat and depending on your specific body composition, we can survive off of this energy for long periods of time - Fasting.

FASTING

Fasting is the action of purposely abstaining from foods or anything that causes or creates an insulin spike. This has been practiced by various cultures for centuries and is done for various reasons and different durations, including religious, spirituality, health and weight management.

Examples of religious or spiritual fasting would be Ramadan fasting in Islam, Yom Kippur fasting in Judaism and Lenten fasting in Christianity.

Fasting for weight management can be along the lines of Intermittent Fasting where you are setting aside portions of the day and up to full days without consuming anything - maintaining an 8-hour window for eating or eating every other day.

Interesting to note that the longest documented fast was 382 days by a Scottish man named Angus Barbieri, from June 1965 to July 1966. In doing this, he'd lost 276 pounds while living off of only tea, coffee, soda water and vitamins. Consuming these items may not seem like a true fast but your body can still be in a fasted state while you are taking on more than just water and depending on your size and energy expenditures throughout a day, can even include 50-100 calories.

Fasting for health focuses on prolonged periods of time - days - only consuming water or clear beverages with no sugars - tea, coffee, BROTH and while you are ill, your body may actually be sending you this exact message. As stated under Cachexia, a shift in your appetite-regulating hormones, such as ghrelin - is what is most likely causing your lack of appetite.

Ghrelin: is a hormone produced in your stomach and small intestine and plays a significant role in regulating your appetite, but also physiological processes related to energy balance and metabolism. Under normal circumstances, Ghrelin - referred to as your "hunger hormone", is what is telling your body when it's time to eat, or that you are hungry. In a weakened state, under chronic illness or viral attack, the reason you may not be particularly hungry is because your body is communicating with you, via this hormone, that it's kind of busy dealing with other things and could use a little less of you trying to help it along.

Addition to this is that Ghrelin can also impact your metabolism in that when it's telling you that you are not hungry or after consuming a meal that you are already full, it's also stimulating the utilization of stored fat to help balance your energy requirements.

Listening to our body when our brains have been bombarded by conflicting information has become increasingly more difficult. We rationalize that if we don't eat, we won't have the energy to maintain living function, could possibly die and if you didn't start off at 456 pounds like Angus Barbieri before his over yearlong fast, you might even believe this strong enough to override your body trying to communicate with you. Thing is, Ghrelin also communicates with you by following a Circadian Rhythm (night and day sleep cycles based on your internal clock) so that you are typically not getting up in the middle of the night feeling hungry.

If your body is smart enough to rely on Ghrelin to keep you alive overnight in a period with eating by balancing your energy and toning down your hunger pangs, when you are ill and not feeling hungry, you should pay attention.

In addition to fasting being about weight management, there are a number of other benefits that can come from this practice - whether listening to your body or by conscious decision.

Benefits from Fasting:

Improved Insulin Sensitivity: Fasting may enhance insulin sensitivity, making it easier for the body to regulate blood sugar levels. This can be particularly beneficial for individuals with prediabetes or type 2 diabetes.

Enhanced Fat Burning: During fasting, the body may shift from using glucose as its primary energy source to burning stored fat for fuel. This process, known as ketosis, can promote fat loss.

Autophagy: Fasting can stimulate autophagy, a cellular process that helps remove damaged cells and cellular components. This may have implications for longevity and cellular health.

Reduced Fat Accumulation: Fasting may help reduce the accumulation of fat in the liver. NAFLD is characterized by the accumulation of excess fat in the liver cells, which can lead to inflammation and liver damage. Fasting and calorie restriction can promote the breakdown of stored fat, including in the liver.

Restoring Function to The Pancreas: Fasting gives time to your pancreas to recover and work again for producing insulin and enzymes and is known to cause physiological changes in the endocrine pancreas, including decreased insulin secretion and increased reactive oxygen species (ROS) production.

Reduction in Oxidative Stress: Fasting and intermittent fasting may reduce oxidative stress and inflammation in the body, which can have a protective effect on kidney tissue. Chronic inflammation and oxidative stress are linked to kidney damage.

Cardiovascular Health: Some studies suggest that intermittent fasting may improve cardiovascular risk factors, such as blood pressure, cholesterol levels, and triglycerides.

Inflammation Reduction: Fasting has been associated with reductions in markers of inflammation, which are linked to various chronic diseases.

Brain Health: There is emerging evidence that fasting may support brain health and cognitive function. Some studies suggest that it may enhance brain-derived neurotrophic factor (BDNF), a protein associated with learning and memory.

Longevity: Research on animals has shown that caloric restriction and intermittent fasting can extend lifespan. While the evidence in humans is less clear, fasting's potential impact on aging is an area of ongoing research.

Improved Eating Patterns: Fasting can promote more mindful eating and reduce the tendency to snack throughout the day. It may also help break the cycle of emotional or habitual eating.

Digestive Rest: Fasting gives the digestive system a break from processing food, which some people find refreshing and may provide temporary relief from gastrointestinal issues.

And specific to being ill, your body will benefit from a fast through the reduction of inflammation, autophagy, and vital organ function.

Having covered eating inflammatory foods or spiking your immune response with higher glycemic foods and fillers, one thing that you may already understand is that these are not permanent effects. Simply not eating these for any period of time, your body will digest/metabolize them, store the excess energy and expel the waste. The benefit from just not having these will be the inverse effect of consumption - reduce inflammatory triggering, minimize the cytokine response and preserve immune energy for where it's actually needed.

Autophagy, which means "Self-Eating", in Greek, is much the same as the previously stated digestive/metabolism process but more internal. While this process occurs continuously in our bodies, it has a more profound impact during a fasted state. The body isn't actually eating itself in a way that can cause additional damages, what it is doing is recycling old and damaged cells for use as nutrients. The dysfunctional cells that it works to clear out may be the body's source of internal injury or the cause of inflammation inside of the body. Removing these damaged cells also works to preserve immune energy for where and when it's actually needed.

In a fasted state, your body will still require energy and immune energy and with your body storing energy in fat and muscle storing immune energy, both seem to be covered. While your muscle stores may be adequate to carry you throughout a fasting period in addition to this, fasting works to improve function of vital organs that have the ability to create creatine. For this process, your body can break down muscles and tissues for their building blocks to generate creatine in your liver, kidneys, and pancreas. The added benefits of fasting is that it can reduce the load on your liver by helping clear it out and deal with stored fat, reduce oxidative stress and improve kidney function as well as has the ability to help regenerate your pancreas.

As many positive benefits that can come from fasting - reduction of inflammation, reduced load on vital organs, clearing out damaged cells, there is one negative impact that you may suffer from and not a welcomed impact if you are already under the weather.

The Keto Flu!

Keto Flu

The "keto flu" refers to a set of symptoms that some people experience when they first start a ketogenic diet or a very low-carbohydrate diet. These symptoms typically occur within the first few days to a week of starting the diet as your body adapts to a state of ketosis, where it primarily burns fat for fuel instead of carbohydrates. The keto flu is not an actual illness, but rather a collection of temporary side effects that some individuals may encounter. Common symptoms of the keto flu include:

Fatigue: Feeling unusually tired or lethargic is one of the most common symptoms. As your body adjusts to using ketones for energy instead of carbohydrates, you may experience a drop in energy levels.

Headache: Some people report experiencing headaches during the initial stages of a ketogenic diet. This could be due to changes in electrolyte balance and fluid retention.

Nausea: Nausea or an upset stomach may occur as your digestive system adapts to the dietary changes. Some individuals may also experience digestive discomfort.

Dizziness and Lightheadedness: A drop in blood sugar levels, dehydration, or changes in blood pressure can lead to feelings of dizziness or lightheadedness.

Irritability and Mood Swings: Changes in blood sugar and hormone levels can affect mood and lead to irritability, anxiety, or mood swings.

Difficulty Sleeping: Some people may have trouble sleeping or experience changes in their sleep patterns when they first start a ketogenic diet.

Muscle Cramps: Electrolyte imbalances, particularly a reduction in sodium and potassium, can lead to muscle cramps.

Brain Fog: You might have trouble concentrating or thinking clearly, often referred to as "brain fog."

All of these symptoms can already be present with your viral infection, but they may in fact get a little worse once your body has been deprived of carbohydrates/sugars and switches into using Ketones - Fat - for Energy. The best thing that you can do to mitigate these conditions is to consume…

[Chicken Broth has entered the conversation]

Early on in covering the benefits from the vitamin profiles of each of the ingredients, I'd mentioned that having these combined makes up an excellent electrolytic profile, has no added chemicals, colors, flavor or sugars and if you've ever had the Keto Flu, is the best thing you can do to remedy the bulk of these symptoms. Addition to this, if you've used the skin in your soup, you will get an added blast of healthy fats to help clear up muddled thoughts and provide a little punch of energy.

Less is More.

While I have openly admitted that you are only getting trace amounts of vitamins, minerals, nutrients, and amino acids, you are getting some. These small amounts can provide your body with the relief it needs from symptoms of the Keto Flu and while still only miniscule in quantities, it is important to realize the Net Nutritional Value Effect.

Net value is something we all have some sense of.

Ex. Your Gross Salary - Taxes = Net Income.

Applied to food:

Food Value - Inflammatory Ingredients = Net Nutritional Value

We all like to see the largest Net Nutritional Value possible, but what if I told you that this number could actually be a negative value and especially with consumption of processed and fast foods?

Not that French Fries or Potatoes are great quality food choices, I'm going to use them as an example to break this down.

What is the Nutritional Value of a Medium French Fries?
320 Cal
15g Fats
43g Carbs

Ingredients: Potato, **Vegetable Oil (canola Oil, Corn Oil, Soybean Oil, Hydrogenated Soybean Oil, Natural Beef Flavor [wheat And Milk Derivatives]),   Dextrose,   Sodium   Acid Pyrophosphate (maintain Color), Salt. *Natural Beef Flavor Contains Hydrolyzed Wheat and Hydrolyzed Milk as Starting Ingredients.**

What is the Nutritional Value of a Potato?
91 Cal
.11g Fats
22g Carbs

Ingredients: Potato.

When you consider that there isn't a single additional ingredient that goes into making French Fries that adds Nutritional Value, what you have to do is appreciate the fact that taking 114g of potatoes and making them into fries, you are going to see 3.5x the Calories, 136x the fat content and double the carb load. Any actual value besides being a belly filler is completely lost.

You'll find the same with turning a quarter pound of hamburger into a QP with cheese (Dr. James H. Salisbury is rolling over in his grave over this). By the time you've added the bun and condiments, and while you haven't erased some nutritional quality, you've neutralized the impact. As for others... Pizza? Lasagna? Spaghetti? Chicken Nuggets? Muffins? Donuts? Biscuits? Pancakes? Waffles? All the same.

Yes. We all know that processed and fast foods aren't great and are probably not the foods you want to take on when you're fighting off the sniffles, now maybe a better understanding as to why. The point is to show that even in trace quantities consuming food with a Net Positive Food Value, Less can actually be More.

4200+ words and 30(ish) pages to make that point.

I hope you appreciate this effort as much as I appreciate your patience in making it through to this point.

Let's bring it all together now.

Conclusion

Chicken Soup can be served as a hearty soup to provide a wide variety of vitamins, minerals, nutrients, and amino acids, to support your immune health, immune energy, reduce oxidative stress and to help keep you warm on a cold day.

As a broth, it serves as a low glycemic beverage rich in electrolytes and through net positive nutritional values, it still supports immune function while working to reduce inflammation and symptoms that may be brought on in a viral fasting state.

There is a lot more information available today than would have been for Hippocrates in the 5th Century BCE on the immune system, functions of the body and the impacts of food. With this being said, his consideration of letting food be thy medicine seems to still hold true today as would his prescription for Chicken Soup as a therapeutic during a respiratory virus.

References:

PubMed - information on Sarcopenia, Cachexia, and various studies for information on benefits of vitamins, minerals, nutrients and amino acids, thermogenesis, ATP, autophagy

Examine.com - information on benefits of vitamins, minerals, nutrients, and amino acid

Wikipedia - information on vitamins, minerals, nutrients, immune triggers

Mcdonalds.ca - breakdown of nutritional information and ingredients - nuggets and fries

Thezebra.com - information on antidepressants

Cihi.ca - information on antidepressants, antipsychotics, benzos - re: seniors

NHS - most common side effects of antidepressants

Medical News Today - most common side effects of pharmaceuticals

Mayo Clinic - RDA for vitamins, common symptoms of Long COVID

Healthline - Benefits of fasting, autophagy keto flu, thermogenesis, piperine,

Cleaveland Clinic – Autophagy, immune system
NIH – Immune triggers

Dedication to the Veterans from our small but global reaching community:

Donations to Veterans Food Banks, globally, have been made by members from our community as well as proceeds from the book will also be extended. A universal message from those who were able to give, those in our community who've supported and continue to support this effort and myself:

To Our Beloved Veterans,

In honor of your unwavering courage and service to our nations, we've dedicated this tribute to you. Your sacrifices have paved the way for our freedoms, and your bravery continues to inspire us all.

As we dedicate this gesture to our veterans, we promise to remember, honor, and support you always.

Your legacy of service lives on, and your sacrifices will forever be etched in our hearts.

With profound respect and heartfelt gratitude,

The YakkStack Community.

www.ingramcontent.com/pod-product-compliance
Lightning Source LLC
Chambersburg PA
CBHW071710020426
42333CB00017B/2211